General Pathology, Microbiology and Immu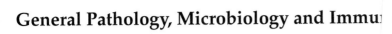

Illustrator: Robert Britton

For Churchill Livingstone:

Commissioning Editor: Ellen Green
Project Manager: Valerie Burgess
Project Development Editor: Mairi McCubbin
Designer: Judith Wright
Copy-editor: Colin Nicholls
Indexer: Jill Halliday
Page Layout: Kate Walshaw
Sales promotion executive: Hilary Brown

General Pathology, Microbiology and Immunology

for Health Care Students

J. H. L. Playfair MB BChir PhD DSc

Emeritus Professor, Dept of Immunology,
University College London Medical School,
London

P. M. Lydyard MSc PhD

Professor, Department of Immunology,
University College London Medical School,
London

S. R. Lakhani BSc MBBS MD MRCPath

Senior Lecturer and Honorary Consultant,
Department of Histopathology,
University College London Medical School,
London

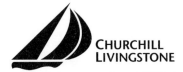
CHURCHILL
LIVINGSTONE

EDINBURGH LONDON NEW YORK PHILADELPHIA SAN FRANCISCO SYDNEY TORONTO 1998

CHURCHILL LIVINGSTONE
Medical Division of Harcourt Brace and Company Limited

© Harcourt Brace and Company Limited 1998

 is a registered trademark of Harcourt Brace and Company Limited

First edition 1998

ISBN 0 443 05722 2

British Library of Cataloguing in Publication Data
A catalogue record for this book is available from the British Library.

Library of Congress Cataloging in Publication Data
A catalogue record for this book is available from the Library of Congress

Medical knowledge is constantly changing. As new information becomes available, changes in treatment, procedures, equipment and the use of drugs become necessary. The editors/authors/contributors and the publishers have, as far as it is possible, taken care to ensure that the information given in this text is accurate and up to date. However, readers are strongly advised to confirm that the information, especially with regard to drug usage, complies with latest legislation and and standards of practice.

The publisher's policy is to use paper manufactured from sustainable forests

Printed and bound in Great Britain at The Bath Press, Bath

Contents

Preface

Many years of teaching and discussion with undergraduate nurses, physiotherapists, podiatrists and radiologists have convinced us that, while a basic understanding of microbiology, immunology and pathology is vital to all health scientists, the available textbooks are either too large or too specialised, or both. In this short book we have tried to provide an essential database on the general area of 'infection, immunity and the response to disease', which is covered in virtually all undergraduate degree courses based on health science.

Each of the 13 chapters is introduced by one or more clinical cases, with emphasis on features of interest to individual disciplines, suggestions for addional reading, and a self-test section in the form of typical essay questions with suggested answers. Additional useful information will be found in the four appendices and glossary of technical terms.

We have assumed a basic knowledge of the working of the normal body, as covered, for example, in Sigrid Rutishauser's excellent *Physiology and Anatomy: a Basis for Nursing and Health Care*[1], and we hope that our book will, in turn, lead on to the more specialised clinical texts required by the various health care professions.

We would like to express our gratitude to all those teachers and students who helped us clarify our ideas for the book, and in particular Barbara Banks, David Bender, Martin Collins, David Flinton, David Maskell, Frances O' Brien and Barbara Wall.

London 1997

J.H.L. Playfair
P.M. Lydyard
S.R. Lakhani

---

[1] Rutishauser S 1994 Physiology and anatomy: a basis for nursing and health care. Churchill Livingstone, Edinburgh

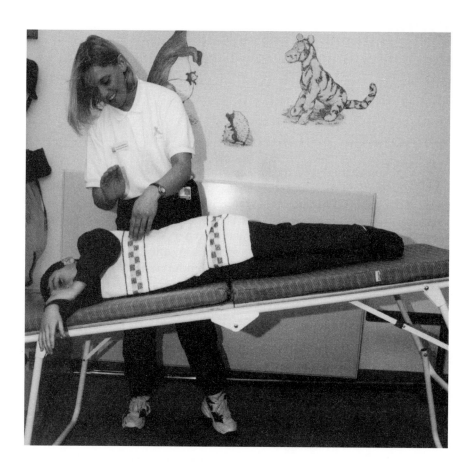

A seven-year-old boy receiving physiotherapy to help him bring up unusually sticky sputum – one consequence of the disease cystic fibrosis. In this opening chapter we consider the broad roles of genetic and environmental factors in this and many other conditions, with an emphasis on the part played by microbial infection and immune mechanisms, which are discussed in detail in the rest of the book.

(Reproduced with kind permission from Birmingham Heartlands Hospital.)

Genes and environment

1

Case 1.1
Now 7, Chris is small for his age, and while the other boys go to play football he has to have physiotherapy for his chest. Chris also receives extracts of a pancreatic enzyme to stop him getting diarrhoea and he also has to take regular multivitamin supplements each day.

From the above information, it is difficult to arrive at a precise diagnosis, but a number of questions should come to mind. Why does Chris need pancreatic enzyme and vitamin supplements? Presumably he cannot make his own enzyme, which means he has pancreatic insufficiency. The physiotherapy to his chest is to help him to bring up sputum – but why cannot he do this himself? The answer is that it is unusually sticky, and when it was cultured recently the microbiologist reported 'a heavy growth of *Pseudomonas aeruginosa*'. His last X-ray showed 'bronchial dilatation' (bronchiectasis). This is an unusual scenario involving a rare type of bacterium, and prompts further questions. Is his resistance to infection impaired? Should an immunologist be consulted? Is the infection contagious? A clue might come from other family members. But his father and mother and his one sister are quite normal, which appears to rule out an inherited condition too – or does it? To begin to understand and manage Chris's condition, some knowledge of the lungs and the pancreas, of bacteria and immunity, of inheritance, and of treatment are evidently needed.

In fact, Chris's condition is inherited, because both his parents carry the gene for *cystic fibrosis*. The disease is inherited in an autosomal recessive fashion, which means that for the person to be affected he has to have two defective copies of the gene – one from each parent. The person with the two defective copies is referred to as being *homozygous* for the gene. Both the parents are *heterozygous* – i.e. they each carry only one defective copy and it is for this reason that they are clinically normal. The one normal copy of the gene is sufficient to avert the symptoms of cystic fibrosis. Cystic fibrosis is a widespread disorder that affects many of the secretory processes in the body and the affected organs include lungs, pancreas, liver, bowel, salivary glands and testis. The basic defect is an inability to regulate the chloride ion transport across cell membranes, which leads to abnormalities of secretions in body spaces. In the lung, for instance, this leads to thick, viscous mucus being produced, which is difficult to clear and leads to blockage of bronchi and eventually a pneumonia behind the obstruction. Similarly, the blockage of pancreatic ducts leads to obstruction and destruction of parts of the pancreas, which leads to reduction in the enzymes that are needed for fat absorption in the bowel. When this is extensive, replacements have to be given, as in Chris's case. Since fat absorption is also vital to the absorption of certain vitamins, supplements of these may also have to be included in the daily routine. The liver, bowel, and testes can be affected too by this inability to regulate the chloride ions.

Cystic fibrosis is therefore a *genetic* disease, caused by a single abnormal gene. The gene has been located on chromosome 7 (band q31–32). In keeping with the clinical findings, the gene has been shown to encode a protein that acts as a chloride channel. The incidence is approximately 1 in 2000 live births and it has been estimated that as many as one person in 20 may be a carrier (i.e. heterozygous) in some populations.

The lung infection is caused by bacteria coming from outside – an *environmental* contribution. The thick mucus in the bronchi prevents the removal of bacteria from the airways. Initially this is intermittent, but eventually it becomes a chronic infection, leading to tissue destruction and permanent dilatations of the peripheral bronchi (bronchiectasis). It is this interaction of genetic and environmental factors that make Chris's life such a misery.

In this chapter we shall show how all disease can be traced ultimately to these two factors – genes and environment – operating sometimes in isolation but frequently together (Table 1.1). We shall first look at some common

Table 1.1 The causes of disease can be classified into genetic (or inborn) and environmental (or acquired)

Genetic	
DNA	Mutations
Chromosome	Lost or extra chromosomes
	Breakage (deletion, translocation, insertion)
Multifactorial	e.g. malformations

Environmental	
Physical	Injury (heat, cold, trauma)
Chemical	Drugs, poisons
Deficiencies	Oxygen, calories, protein, vitamins
Microbial	Viruses, bacteria, etc.
Immunological[1]	Hypersensitivities
Psychological[1]	Psychoses, neuroses

[1] *May be genetic contribution as well.*

genetic disorders. On the environmental side, we shall consider briefly the effect of physical and chemical injury, and of deficiencies of essential requirements, before focusing on the microbes that cause infectious disease and the ways the body defends itself against them, introducing the study of *microbiology* and *immunology*. In the following chapter we shall describe the ways in which cells and tissues react to these various noxious agents – the study of *histopathology*. In later chapters you will see that, though usually taught as separate subjects, microbiology, immunology, and histopathology are so closely interlinked that a basic understanding of all three disciplines is often needed in order to understand what is wrong with a particular patient.

GENETIC DISEASE

Genes are those portions of an individual's DNA that code for his proteins, the equivalent of a blueprint for his construction and function. It has been known since the days of Watson and Crick that DNA carries the *genetic code*, based on the four bases – guanine, adenine, thymine and cytosine. The sequence of these bases is used as a template to synthesize messenger RNA (mRNA) by complementary base pairing ('transcription'). The mRNA then leaves the nucleus and associates with ribosomes in the cytoplasm. There, individual triplets of bases in a sequence in the mRNA, known as *codons*, pair with complementary triplets on transfer RNA (tRNA) molecules which are linked to different amino acids (see Fig. 1.1).

Differences in genes are responsible for the normal differences between people – height, eye colour, blood group, etc. However, in some genes, a difference from the normal can cause an obvious abnormality, which may range from the merely inconvenient (e.g. colour blindness) to the serious or life-threatening (e.g. haemophilia, cystic fibrosis). These differences may consist of a single changed base, causing a single changed amino acid in some vital protein (e.g. the β chain of haemoglobin in sickle cell disease; see Fig. 1.1), or they may be a result of a whole extra chromosome being present. This would mean having an enormous amount of extra DNA, with its hundreds of genes, and this is easily identifiable in a microscope preparation (e.g. chromosome 21 in Down's syndrome; see Fig. 1.2). Some genetic diseases, such as cystic fibrosis, appear to be due to abnormalities of a *single* gene. Many other diseases that 'run in families', including well-known congenital malformations such as spina bifida, are clearly of genetic origin, but *multiple* genes are probably involved and these have not been identified. In cystic fibrosis, the presence of two abnormal copies of the gene means a 100% certainty of having the manifestations of the disease. However, there are many situations where genetic alterations produce a *predisposition* rather than an absolute certainty. For example, inheriting a mutation in the breast cancer susceptibility gene *BRCA1* means an 80% lifetime risk of getting breast cancer, and abnormalities of the Ataxia-telangiectasia gene also predispose to breast cancer, but in a smaller proportion of cases. These predisposing genetic events sometimes only become significant if the right environmental factors are also present. These may

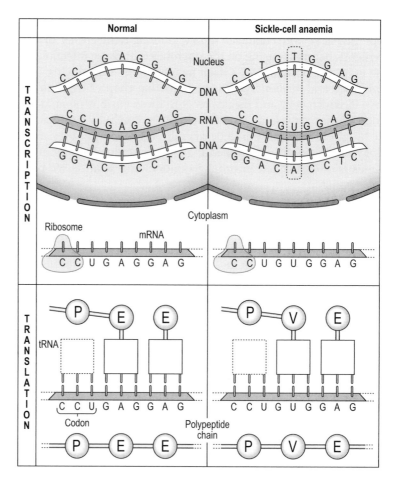

Fig. 1.1 How a point mutation in the DNA coding for the β-globin chain of haemoglobin on chromosome 11 can lead to an alteration in the amino acid sequence. Note that in the sickle cell gene, a mutation of an adenine (A) to a thymine (T) in the triplet coding for glutamic acid in the DNA gives rise to a valine instead. This alteration in the β-globin amino acid sequence leads to a functional change in the properties of haemoglobin and 'sickling' of the red blood cells in unusual situations of hypoxia. The problem is most severe in homozygotes, while patients with only one affected chromosome (heterozygotes) suffer only occasionally, since they also have normal haemoglobin coded for by the other chromosome. This form of anaemia will be discussed in more detail in a later chapter. The single letter code for amino acids is used here: P, proline; E, glutamic acid; V, valine.

show up quite late in life, a good example being atherosclerosis. See Table 1.2 for a list of the most important conditions in these various categories.

Inheritance patterns

Within classical genetics and molecular genetics, there is an overlap of terminology which often causes confusion. We have already discussed types of inheritance in considering the example of cystic fibrosis. This is an autosomal recessive disorder, meaning that two abnormal copies of the gene have to be present to produce disease. The person having cystic fibrosis

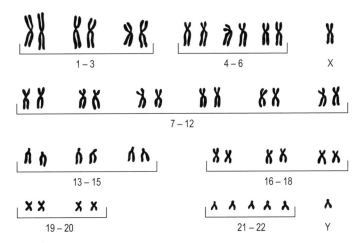

Fig. 1.2 Karyotype in Down's syndrome, showing three no. 21 chromosomes instead of the normal two. (Courtesy of Professor M.A. Ferguson-Smith.)

is then *homozygous* for the gene. The parents who each contributed one abnormal gene are *heterozygous* for the gene and are *carriers* since they do not have the manifestations of the disease. This type of disease is much more common in those who intermarry, since they are much more likely to carry one copy of the same abnormal gene. Hence, autosomal recessive disorders are common in certain groups – e.g. Muslims – who regularly marry within the family. Interestingly, cystic fibrosis is common within the white population but is distinctly uncommon amongst Asian and black populations.

In contrast, an autosomal dominant disorder is one which manifests when only one abnormal gene is present, showing that the presence of one normal copy (allele) does not prevent the disease. It is not possible therefore to be a carrier for such a disorder, and an affected individual will have a 1 in 2 chance of passing the gene on to his children. Examples are polycystic kidney and familial hypercholesterolaemia.

In *sex-linked* inheritance, the disease-producing gene is located on the X-chromosome. In the female, the presence of one normal and one abnormal X-chromosome does not produce disease and the female is a carrier. This is therefore a special type of recessive disorder. In men, the inheritance of the abnormal X-chromosome from their mother leads to disease, since the second sex chromosome in men is a Y-chromosome. Sex-linked disorders are therefore generally carried by females and transmitted to males who express the disease. Women are only affected in the rare case of an affected male having a female child with a carrier female. A good example of a sex-linked disorder is haemophilia (see Figs 1.3 and 1.4).

Mutations – dominant and recessive

Very simply, a mutation is an alteration in the base sequence of the DNA. These alterations can take a number of forms. They may be a result of a *point mutation*, which means a change in one base pair, as occurs in sickle

Table 1.2 The major genetic diseases

Single gene mutations	
Haemoglobinopathies	Sickle cell disease, thalassaemia
Aminoacidopathies	Phenylketonuria, alkaptonuria Homocystinuria, G6P deficiency
Immunodeficiencies Haemochromatosis Cystic fibrosis Polyposis coli Familial hypercholesterolaemia Haemophilia Polycystic kidney Colour blindness Albinism Duchenne muscular dystrophy	(Several)
Chromosome abnormalities	
Extra chromosome	Down's syndrome (extra 21) Klinefelter's syndrome (extra X) Edwards' syndrome (extra 18) Patau's syndrome (extra 13)
Missing chromosome	Turner's syndrome (missing X; i.e. XO)
Breakage/translocation	Burkitt's lymphoma (8–2, 14, 22) Chronic myeloid leukaemia (9–22)
Polygenic and/or multifactorial	
Cleft palate Club foot Congenital heart disease Congenital dislocation of hip Pyloric stenosis Spina bifida	
Predisposition to	Atherosclerosis Allergy Diabetes Epilepsy Thyroiditis Tumours

cell disease. In this particular case the point mutation is *intragenic*, meaning inside the coding region of the gene, and is therefore likely to have an effect on the protein and hence the function of that gene. A point mutation occurring in the non-coding region may not have any significant effect clinically. Mutations may also be large and involve loss of many genes or whole chromosomes, and these are called *deletions*. Genetic material may be transferred from one chromosome and come to lie on another chromosome and this is called *translocation* or *rearrangement*. In some instances, the gene is multiplied many hundreds of times, so that, instead of one copy, numerous copies are present within the segment of DNA. This is called *amplification*.

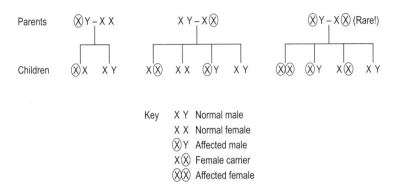

Key
X Y Normal male
X X Normal female
ⓍY Affected male
XⓍ Female carrier
ⓍⓍ Affected female

Fig. 1.3 In sex-linked diseases such as haemophilia, three patterns of inheritance can occur. In these hypothetical families, the X chromosome carrying the mutation is shown circled.

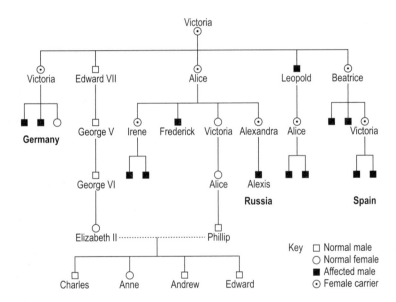

Key □ Normal male
○ Normal female
■ Affected male
⊙ Female carrier

Fig. 1.4 Haemophilia was widespread in the royal families of Europe descended from Queen Victoria, who was a carrier. Fortunately the present British royal family, despite a marriage between fourth cousins, does not carry the gene for haemophilia.

A confusion in terminology sometimes occurs because the terminology of molecular genetics has been borrowed from inheritance genetics. For example, cancer-producing genes called *oncogenes* have been divided into two types; dominant oncogenes and recessive oncogenes (better called tumour suppressor genes). These are dealt with in Chapter 12, but we will mention them briefly here to illustrate the confusion that may arise because of the terminology. In the former, mutation in one copy of the gene (one allele) leads to a predisposition to cancer; hence they are called 'dominant' or 'gain in function' mutations. In recessive oncogenes, both alleles have to be inactivated to remove the inhibition to tumour formation and allow tumour growth, so these are called 'recessive' or 'loss of function' mutations. A further confusion occurs because with some genetic predispositions to cancer, e.g. the BRCA1 gene for breast cancer, mutation in one allele which is inherited from the parent produces a dominant inheritance pattern to the predisposition. However, for the disease to occur, the second copy also has to undergo mutation, since the gene is a recessive oncogene (tumour suppressor gene). So, confusingly, the patient has a dominant inheritance susceptibility but a recessive action at a genetic level.

The above may make you think that mutations are a bad thing. This is not necessarily so. You may not realize it, but if mutations did not happen, you would not be reading this book. Actually we would not have written it in the first place!

If you imagine a piece of string that has acquired the ability to replicate itself precisely, you can imagine that, after replication, you would not be able to tell which was the original piece of string. If this went on for a thousand years, you would still have string being produced which was identical to its parent. But if in the replication a mistake was made, then things would become interesting. Let us imagine, for instance, that the mistake leads to the string becoming blue instead of white. If the mistake only occurred rarely, you would still have many white pieces and the odd blue one. If a further mistake in the copying leads the blue to become red, in time a number of red ones will also appear. Of course you can see that the proportions of each type will depend on the time and the frequency of the mistake in copying. This is fundamentally what evolutionary mutations are about. Our genetic machinery is so sophisticated that, despite thousands of replications in a lifetime, very few mistakes are made. Most of those that are made are corrected very efficiently by an array of repair mechanisms. But a few mutations do persist, and if these occur in 'germ' cells (sperm or ova) they can be passed to the next generation, and over millions of years subtle changes begin to show in the species. So evolution is a very slow process, but, without these mistakes in the copying, we would not exist in our present form. Evolutionary theory states that besides these mistakes, there has to be a 'pressure for survival'. Mutational changes are random, and many will confer a disadvantage and probably die out in time. Those that are advantageous will survive and spread. Sickle cell disease is an excellent example of a disease-causing mutation which has probably been allowed to survive because of its usefulness. In an area infested with malaria, having one sickle cell mutation confers a survival advantage, since red cells infected with the parasite will sickle and die. However, as the mutation spreads in the community, people who have this beneficial mutation will meet and marry, and hence produce children who carry two mutations. Now their cells sickle not only with malaria but also under conditions of low oxygen, producing life-threatening events, the sickle crises – a definite disadvantage. This balance of advantage and disadvantage tends to keep the proportions of the normal and the sickle gene fairly stable in a population, a condition known as 'balanced polymorphism'.

ENVIRONMENTAL DISORDERS

Physical injury

Wounding, burning, and freezing cause direct destruction of tissues and their effects are usually visible. But invisible forms of energy can also be highly dangerous, examples being electric shock and radiation sickness. The main effect of ionizing radiation (e.g. X-rays) is damage to DNA, and this is particularly insidious because with certain doses symptoms may not appear for a week or more, as the stoppage of new blood cell production in the bone marrow gradually leads to infections and bleeding disorders. Later, as the atomic bomb on Hiroshima made all too evident, various cancers may appear. Electric shock, on the other hand, mainly affects the heart, and if resuscitation is successful and there is no burning, there should be no after-effects.

Chemical injury

Chemicals may be definitely poisonous (e.g. cyanide, arsenic), essentially harmless (e.g. food additives), or intended to do good (e.g. therapeutic drugs). Unfortunately these categories overlap somewhat, and this is particularly important when considering the harmful side-effects of drugs, which are seen mainly in two situations: (i) with *overdoses* (e.g. barbiturate poisoning) and (ii) when an individual patient is *hypersensitive* to a normal dose of a drug (e.g. penicillin allergy).

Deficiency diseases

Worldwide, malnutrition is probably the commonest cause of ill-health, with millions of our fellow men and women still literally starving to death. But even a diet adequate in calories can be lacking in particular essentials such as protein, iron, vitamins, iodine, and 'trace' metals such as zinc and copper. One should also remember that excessive intake of some food components can predispose to disease – alcohol, salt, sugar, and saturated fats being well-publicized examples. Remember, too, that in addition to the direct effects of alcohol, mainly on the liver and brain, alcoholics frequently have a diet deficient in vitamins. Another element vital to life is, of course, oxygen, but this, too, can be extremely toxic in excess; indeed, many of the effects of radiation, and perhaps even normal ageing, are thought to be due to the production of *free radicals* from oxygen. Table 1.3 lists the commoner deficiency conditions and their consequences.

Microbial disease

This is virtually synonymous with infection – though, strictly speaking, microbes (or microorganisms) are those transmissible disease agents that you need a microscope to see: namely viruses, bacteria, smaller fungi, and protozoa. However, some visible organisms, such as large fungi and worms, cause disease in just the same way, so *infectious disease* is a better term, and will be used throughout this book. But, for convenience, the agents themselves will all be referred to as *microorganisms*.

Table 1.3 Common deficiencies and their main consequences

Calories (i.e. energy)	Weight loss, growth retardation
Protein	Weight loss, oedema (kwashiorkor)
Iron	Anaemia
Iodine	Goitre (swollen thyroid), cretinism
Zinc, copper	Immunodeficiency, skin rashes
Oxygen	Respiratory failure
Vitamins	
A	Night blindness, immunodeficiency
B_1 (thiamine)	Peripheral neuropathy, beriberi
B_2 (riboflavin)	Dry mouth, anaemia
Niacin	Pellagra
B_6 (pyridoxine)	Dry skin, neuropathy
B_{12} (cobalamine)	Pernicious anaemia
Folate	Pernicious anaemia
C (ascorbic acid)	Scurvy
D	Rickets (children), osteomalacia (adults)
E	Anaemia, neuropathy (rare)
K	Bleeding

Details of the organisms and how they cause disease will be found in Chapters 3 and 4; here we will merely point out that, as the case of Chris illustrates, there is often a contribution by the patient to an infectious disease. He may have a gross defect in some defence mechanism, as Chris does in his lungs; his resistance may be weakened by dietary deficiency, radiation, or drug treatment, or by another disease such as diabetes or cancer; or he may be unusually susceptible to a particular infection because of an inherited tendency whose genetic basis has not yet been worked out. Very few microorganisms cause exactly the same disease in everyone, and sometimes the effects of exposure to the same dose of infection can range all the way from no symptoms at all to death. These genetic differences are probably 'built in' to successful species of animals to reduce the chance of some newly emerging infection wiping them out altogether.

Immunological disease

Immunological diseases are some of the most surprising. As Chapters 5 and 6 will explain, the immune system is designed expressly to combat infectious disease, all of its many functions being related to killing or otherwise inhibiting microorganisms. So why should it cause disease? The answer is that, like any other complex system – the nervous system, for example – the immune system can over-react or act inappropriately. Details of the ways in which this can happen, and their consequences (usually referred to as *immunopathology*), will be found in Chapter 7; they include common conditions such as allergies, and many important diseases of the skin, kidney, and endocrine organs. The immune system can also under-react, which leads, as you would expect, to an increased susceptibility to infection – a situation known as *immunodeficiency*.

One of the great virtues of the immune system is that – again, like the nervous system – it displays *memory*, it can literally learn to cope better with repeated attacks of the same infection. This is why it is nowadays possible to protect people against (some) infectious diseases by *vaccination* – a form of medical treatment which goes back at least 200 years, but which was not really understood until the development of modern immunology.

MULTIFACTORIAL DISORDERS

Psychological disease

For completeness, we should also mention those conditions in which it is difficult to dissect out precisely the role of either genetics or environmental factors in disease causation. This would include examples such as the psychoses (e.g. schizophrenia) and neuroses (depression, anxiety etc.), for which at present there is no satisfactory physical explanation. It is quite clear that many physical illnesses for which there is ample proof of genetic or environmental aetiology can affect the mental state. Thyroid diseases due to whatever cause can have a profound effect on the mental state of the patient, ranging from marked overactivity in thyrotoxicosis to severe depression in hypothyroidism. In the reverse situation, there is now increasing evidence for molecular links between the nervous, endocrine, and immune systems, which is beginning to put on a firmer footing the popular idea that, for example, stress or depression can influence one's resistance to infection.

Tutorial 1

A good way to test your understanding of a topic is to write short essays (you will have to do this in your exams anyway!). Make notes of what you would include in a 30-minute answer to each of the following questions, which are based on the chapter you have just read, and then compare them with the specimens on the next page. Remember: there is no single 'right' answer to an essay question, but you should include at least some correct facts, plus some interesting discussion. In a science course, you are expected to *think* as well as to *remember*.

QUESTIONS

1. What is a mutation? Why are some mutations more harmful than others?

2. Name three conditions caused by missing or extra chromosomes.

3. Oxygen is both essential to life and toxic. Explain.

4. We all breathe more or less the same air, yet some people constantly get respiratory infections and others never do. Speculate why this might be. (Note: this is an example of a question where at this point you probably know only a few of the relevant facts, but this should not stop you coming up with intelligent suggestions. And in the process you will appreciate why you need to read the rest of this book!)

ANSWERS

1. A mutation is an alteration in the base sequence of the DNA. It may occur in one of the 'non-coding' regions such as the *introns* present in many genes. It may not affect the coding instructions of the base triplet concerned; for example, a change in the RNA from CCU to CCC, CCA, or CCG will not change the coding for proline. Even if the mutation does change an amino acid, this may not have any effect on the function of the corresponding protein. In all these cases, the mutation will be harmless or 'silent'. Remember also that very occasionally a mutation turns out to be beneficial, and that mutations in the germ-line – that is, in the ova or sperm and therefore inherited – are the basis for the evolution of all species.

2. Consult Table 1.2 for the five commonest of these conditions. The commonest of all is Down's syndrome, whose incidence increases with maternal age. There are also some other rare examples of extra sex chromosomes, such as XYY, XXX, XXXY, which show up as abnormal sexual or growth development and often reduced intelligence. True hermaphroditism, with both male and female organs, is extremely rare, and is not associated with any one chromosome pattern.

3. Mammalian respiration depends, of course, on taking up oxygen from the atmosphere and transferring it to the tissues via the red cells of the blood, so that it can be used for *aerobic respiration* in the mitochondria. However, in anaerobic organisms, such as many primitive bacteria, oxygen is actually toxic, and higher animals take advantage of this fact by generating highly toxic molecules derived from oxygen – the so-called *free radicals* – which they use to kill bacteria and fungi. This activity is particularly prominent in a type of phagocytic cell known as the *neutrophil*. Unfortunately, these free radicals, if produced in excess, can also damage the tissues of the host, and they are thought to be responsible for some degenerative conditions such as arteriosclerosis. *Antioxidants* such as vitamins C and E are believed to be able to counteract this, which is why such a range of them are on the market.

4. This question raises the important issue of *susceptibility* to infection, which clearly varies from person to person. Sometimes the reason is known: for example, the individual may be immunodeficient, because of either some developmental failure in his immune system or (more often) some other condition, such as malnutrition, diabetes, cancer, or another underlying infection such as HIV. Occasionally it works the other way: for instance, people carrying the sickle cell gene are actually more *resistant* to malaria. No doubt there are many other genes that confer resistance or susceptibility to particular infections, but which remain to be discovered. Of course, there is also the obvious point that not everybody is exposed to identical microbes: if someone in your house has tuberculosis or you travel in a bus where everyone is coughing and sneezing, you are more *likely* to get infected.

FURTHER READING

Much more detail on the content of this and the following chapter can be found in pathology textbooks. Some examples worth consulting are:

Lakhani S R, Dilly S A, Finlayson C F 1993 Basic pathology. Arnold, London
A lively, amusing and user-friendly book, mainly aimed at medical students.

Mitchinson M J, Arno J, Edwards P A W, LePage R W F, Minson A C 1996 Essentials of pathology. Blackwell Science, Oxford, 346 pp
An excellent new book based on the Cambridge medical course, covering pathology, immunology, and some microbiology, with special emphasis on viruses and cancer.

Muir's textbook of pathology, 13th edn. 1992. Arnold, London 1245 pp
A firm favourite with medical students for over 70 years, very detailed and well illustrated.

Woolf N 1986 Cell, tissue and disease, 2nd edn. Baillière Tindall, London, 503 pp
A very clearly written textbook of basic pathology, with some immunology.

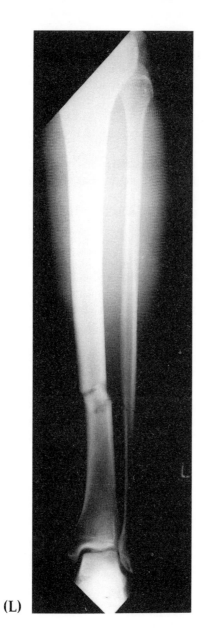
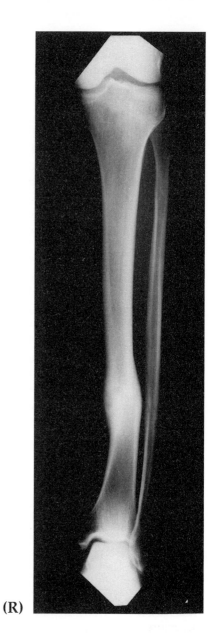

(L)   **(R)**

A 'broken leg' (in fact a compound fracture of the tibia and fibula), immediately after being put in plaster (L) and 18 months later (R). In this chapter we discuss injury and healing of bones and other tissues, with a look at some of the cellular and molecular events that underlie them.

(Reproduced with kind permission from UCL Hospitals NHS Trust, London.)

Cells and tissues: damage and repair

2

■ CONTENTS

Case 2.1

WPC Wendy was stabbed in the arm while arresting a football hooligan who had had too much to drink. She was rushed to hospital and the wound was sterilized and sutured. Her assailant, Mr X, escaped on a motorbike, but crashed and fractured his femur. A week later she was back on duty, but he was in hospital, awaiting surgical exploration of his leg. Why were the outcomes so different?

The body is made up of tissues and organs, which in turn are composed of cells. Disease, however caused (look back to Chapter 1 for a list of causes), can ultimately be traced to the damage or death of cells, although the severity of the disease varies greatly, depending on whether or not the cells can (1) recover or (2) be replaced. In a clean wound, such as Wendy's, thousands of cells may be killed and tissues disrupted, but when the healing process is complete there should be only the faintest scar and no loss of function. Healing of a broken bone also normally restores perfect structure and function, though it takes longer. In both cases, healing can be slowed or prevented by a number of factors including infection, which is probably what happened in X's case. In contrast, damage to the brain, for example because of intracranial bleeding or shortage of oxygen, can lead to permanent disability. The main difference is that dead cells in the skin and subcutaneous tissues can be replaced, while dead brain cells cannot. In fact the skin and the intestines, constantly buffeted by outside forces, are in a permanent state of replacement ('regeneration'), whereas the brain, protected by the hard skull, cannot replace a single one of its hundred thousand million neurones. Table 2.1 compares the regenerative ability of various tissues.

Table 2.1 Regeneration in various cell types

Continuously regenerated	Epithelium (skin, gut, etc.) Bone marrow (blood precursors)
Regenerate only when needed	Fibroblasts, smooth muscle, cartilage, bone Endothelium (blood vessels) Liver, kidney
No regeneration	Neurones Skeletal and heart muscle

CELL INJURY, THE BASIS OF PATHOLOGY

Cells can respond to outside stimuli in several ways. Mild stresses may simply lead to adaptive changes such as increase in size. These types of change are dealt with in Chapter 9. Some stresses are much more severe, and constitute *injury*, from which the cell may either recover or die. The parts of the cell most susceptible to injury are the DNA in the nucleus, the energy source in the mitochondria, the protein-synthesizing ribosomes, and the various membranes that surround the cell and its intracellular structures. Table 2.2 shows that there is a link between different forms of injury and the part of the cell principally affected. It is difficult to say precisely what determines the ability of cells to recover, but evidently each component of the cell has a limit beyond which recovery is impossible, and the cell dies.

The local response to tissue injury is called inflammation and there are two major types: acute and chronic. The differences do not simply lie in the timing. Acute and chronic inflammation have fundamentally different cellular responses and very different clinical outcomes. Let us now consider these in more detail.

Table 2.2 Causes of cell injury and their target

Cause	Main target	Effects on cell or *tissues
Ischaemia (leading to hypoxia)	Mitochondria Ribosomes Lysosomes	Loss of ATP Protein synthesis reduced Cell digests itself *Coagulative necrosis
Free oxygen radicals	Membrane lipids	Lipid peroxidation
Radiation (X-rays; UV)	DNA	Mutations, cancer
Cytotoxic drugs	DNA	Cell division prevented
Antibody + complement	Membrane	Lysis (rupture)
Viruses	Multiply in cell	Lysis
Bacterial toxins	Membranes	Lysis *Liquefactive necrosis (pus)
	Ribosomes	Protein synthesis reduced

INFLAMMATION, HEALING AND REPAIR

Wendy's stab wound would have damaged at least five structures: epidermis, dermis, subcutaneous fat, muscle, and blood vessels, and perhaps some nerves as well. For most of this to be restored to normal in only a few days, events must clearly have moved rapidly. We can distinguish two phases: first an early damage-limiting exercise known as *acute inflammation*, and then the process of *healing and repair* itself.

Acute inflammation

The cardinal signs

Inflammation still means what it meant to the doctors of Roman times – the appearance of a hot, red, painful swelling ('calor, rubor, dolor, tumor') with some loss of normal function – and the changes that bring it about are called the *inflammatory response*. Calor or heat is due to increased blood flow to the inflamed area; rubor (redness) to vascular dilatation, and tumor or swelling to the movement of fluid from the vessels into the surrounding tissues. The mechanisms of dolor or pain are only just beginning to be understood. It is a feature of both acute and, to a lesser extent, chronic inflammation, and often the one that worries the patient most. It is due to stimulation of pain receptors and the nerves that supply them, by a variety of mechanisms, including increased stretching and pressure (e.g. in an abscess or a swollen joint), and molecules released in inflammation (e.g. prostaglandins and prostacyclins). When it warns of the threat of burning or leads to immobilization of an injured or infected part, pain is clearly serving a useful function, but it is hard to see the advantage of, for example, toothache. A curious feature of pain from internal organs is that it is often felt in what seems to be the wrong place ('referred pain'). Thus the anginal pain of cardiac ischaemia commonly occurs in the left arm, and of gall bladder disease in the right shoulder; evidently the brain misreads the stimulus as if it was being transmitted from the body surface by sensory nerves that travel to the same region of the spinal cord as those coming from the organ. The distressing phenomenon of the 'phantom limb' is another example of misinterpretation by the brain. Despite older beliefs to the contrary, it is now considered that young babies feel pain, even though they may be unable to indicate the fact. On the other hand, elderly people are often surprisingly unaware of what would normally be expected to be extremely painful events, such as a heart attack or a fractured bone. Being highly subjective, the perception of pain can be influenced by mental state, suggestion, etc., as well as by the enormous range of pain-killing or *analgesic* drugs. Inevitably, the swelling and pain lead to immobilization of the inflamed tissue and hence loss of function.

Causes of acute inflammation

Since microbial infections are such a common cause of acute inflammation, some of the other causes are easily overlooked. Acute inflammation may also arise as a result of:

- hypersensitivity (allergic) reactions, e.g. secondary to bee stings;
- physical injury;
- radiation injury (X-rays, UV light injury following excessive sunbathing);
- contact with corrosive chemicals;
- vascular injury due to ischaemia.

Inflammation can be unpleasant, and even life-threatening, for example if it leads to breakdown of vital tissue, as can happen when an infected appendix ruptures and spreads the infection into the peritoneal cavity. But it is important to remember that inflammation is basically a protective mechanism, whose function is to clear away damaged tissue and (if present) infectious microorganisms, to try to limit further damage, and to prepare the way for the process of repair.

Regardless of the cause, acute inflammation consists of essentially the same two elements: (1) local response: an increase in blood flow and the passage of blood components from blood to tissues; and (2) systemic response: changes in the production of various mediators that affect distant organs such as the liver and brain. In addition, there may be other early responses to special needs, such as haemostasis to prevent loss of blood.

Local changes: formation of the fluid exudate

Within the body, the normal pressures within the vasculature and the tissues are such that fluid tends to leak out of the arteriolar end of the capillaries and move back in at the venous end. This normal homeostasis is altered during the process of inflammation so that the net effect is a movement of fluid out of the blood vessels and into the tissues. The blood flow and permeability of small blood vessels is affected by a large number of chemical mediators, notably histamine (see Fig. 2.1 for some others). Injury results in the local release of these mediators, resulting in increased blood flow and hence increased pressure which results in leakage of fluid containing potentially useful molecules such as the clotting factors as well as complement and antibody.

The principal sources of the inflammatory mediators are (1) the lipid membranes of damaged cells, (2) mast cells, and (3) the blood plasma. Cell membranes contain arachidonic acid, which can be enzymatically converted to the fatty acid *prostaglandins* and *leukotrienes*, with a whole range of effects on blood vessels and smooth muscle. Anti-inflammatory drugs such as aspirin and indomethacin act mainly to block prostaglandin synthesis. *Mast cells* are particularly interesting; they are prominent in the skin, surrounding blood vessels, and in cavities such as the pleura and peritoneum. The closely similar *basophils* are prominent in the gut and are also present in the blood. Both types of cell contain strikingly dense granules in their cytoplasm, which in turn contain histamine, and are readily released following damage (and also in some allergic conditions; see Chapter 7). This process of mast cell degranulation is the major stimulus to the changes in blood flow mentioned above. From the plasma come the proteins of three important *cascade* systems – so named because they consist of a series of components that activate each other in an amplifying sequence. The clotting system

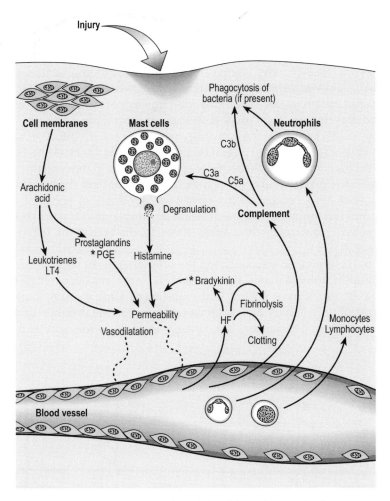

Fig. 2.1 The main changes occurring in the vicinity of tissue damage, leading to acute inflammation. Note that if infection is present, complement, neutrophils, and antibody will help combat this, as described in Chapter 5. HF = Hageman factor (also known as clotting factor XII), an initiator of the kinin, clotting, and fibrinolytic pathways. The components marked with an asterisk are thought to contribute to pain.

is described later (Fig. 2.3); the fibrinolytic system helps to prevent un-controlled clotting, while the kinins contribute to vascular permeability. Figure 2.1 shows the dynamic way in which these various inflammatory pathways interact.

This *inflammatory exudate* is followed shortly by active migration of cells, particularly the mobile phagocytes ('eating cells') known as *neutrophils* (see below).

Formation of the cellular exudate

The cellular elements of the blood normally flow in the centre of the vessels and this type of flow is referred to as laminar flow. During the inflammatory process, the flow becomes sluggish and in some areas may even come to a halt. The cellular elements then come to lie towards the wall of the vessels, and polymorphs (neutrophils), which are the principal cells of acute inflammation, line up adjacent to the endothelial lining. This process is called *margination*. The chemical mediators cause contraction of the endothelial cells and this opens up tiny gaps between the cells. The polymorphs put out projections (pseudopodia) into these tiny gaps and squeeze out into the tissues. This process is termed *emigration*. Later, the polymorphs will be joined by the lymphocytes, whose role in infection will be explained in Chapter 6. The migration of these cells is a fascinating process that involves complex mechanisms of cell adhesion and movement.

Once in the extravascular tissues, the polymorphs find their way to the trouble spot by a process called *chemotaxis*. Products of bacterial membranes and inflammatory mediators such as complement create a gradient of *chemotactic* molecules that guide them to the source of the trouble (see Fig. 2.2).

The polymorphs, on encountering the offending agent such as bacteria, will engulf the foreign material and destroy it by the process of *phagocytosis*. Bacteria are sometimes coated with substances such as complement or immunoglobulins which makes them easier for the neutrophils to recognize and destroy. The process of coating organisms in this way is termed

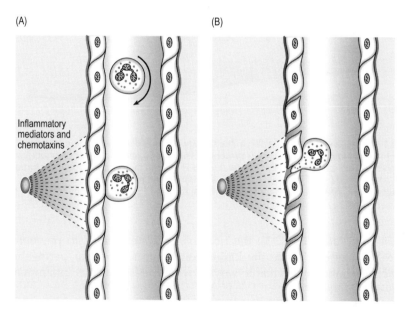

Fig. 2.2 Margination of polymorphs. Damage to blood vessel endothelial cells or surrounding tissue results in the production of inflammatory mediators (e.g. histamine and other molecules like interlukin-1, which induce adhesion molecules on their surface). (A) Polymorphs (PMNs) roll along the endothelial cell surface, slow down, and attach to these molecules (e.g. GMP-140); (B) the mediators also cause contraction of the endothelial cells. Chemotaxins (e.g. complement components at site of bacterial growth) also released in the damaged tissue cause the adhered PMNs to migrate through these intercellular spaces. Once outside the confines of the blood vessel, the PMNs move through a chemotaxin gradient in an 'activated' state, ready to deal with the tissue insult. Platelets and serum proteins also migrate out of the blood vessels to precipitate clotting and tissue repair.

opsonization and the coating substance is called an *opsonin*. Having engulfed them, the phagosome (membrane-bound space in which the bacteria are engulfed) is fused with lysosomes which contain the enzymes needed for the destruction of these foreign particles. Chloride ions and hydrogen peroxide play an important role in this degradation.

Local effects of acute inflammation

These can be divided broadly into (1) beneficial and (2) adverse effects. The beneficial effects include the delivery of antibodies and inflammatory cells to the site of injury and hence the ability to mount an adequate defence response. The same system will of course also deliver drugs such as antibiotics to the site of an infective injury. The production of the fluid exudate will help to dilute any toxins that are produced either by the organisms or by the destruction of tissues following the response.

Adverse effects include tissue destruction, which is a side-effect of the response mounted to combat the injury. Although the response is initiated to protect the body from a 'foreign attack', some degree of self-damage inevitably results. As long as this is not too severe, the body can restore the architecture of these tissues. Occasionally, the swelling resulting from the inflammatory response can itself be life-threatening. An example is epiglottitis in children, which can lead to obstruction of the respiratory tract and asphyxia. Similarly, when swelling occurs in a closed cavity such as during inflammation within the brain, this can lead to a rise in the intracranial pressure which if untreated results in death. Anaphylactic reactions occurring as a result of an allergy to antigen such as pollen or bee sting can also produce a life-threatening inflammatory response.

Systemic effects

Some mediators released during inflammation act at a distance to reset the level of certain body systems. For example, the common occurrence of fever, and even the feeling of 'being ill', are caused by molecules known as cytokines that act on the brain (cytokines, and the cells that make them, will be discussed in Chapter 5). At the same time, the pattern of protein synthesis in the liver is temporarily altered following injury, leading to an increase of several serum proteins involved in damage limitation, and a fall in some others. Those that increase are called *acute phase proteins*, and one of them, C-reactive protein, is often used as a guide to the extent of inflammation – for example in monitoring the course of rheumatic diseases. It is often debated whether fever during inflammation is a good or a bad thing. In infectious diseases a moderate rise of body temperature is probably useful in speeding up inflammatory and immunological processes, and possibly in inhibiting certain microorganisms (malaria-induced fever was once used to treat syphilis for this reason), but very high temperatures above about 41°C (105°F) are in themselves harmful, particularly to the brain. The production of numerous neutrophils from the bone marrow is another example of a systemic response. In severe infections, the ability of the marrow to respond may be overwhelmed, resulting in anaemia and decrease in white blood cell production.

Haemostasis

In circumstances where the vessel wall is damaged directly, as can occur with injury, heat, or cold, three mechanisms go rapidly into action to minimize the loss of blood: (1) small arteries in the vicinity constrict to reduce local blood flow; (2) platelets adhere to the damaged site and attempt to plug the gap; and (3) the process of blood clotting leads to fibrin being deposited, making a more stable and permanent seal (Fig. 2.3). Haemostasis can be defective for many reasons, of which the commonest are a shortage of platelets in the blood (thrombocytopenia) and abnormalities in one of the many clotting factors – deficiency of factor VIII in haemophilia being the best-known.

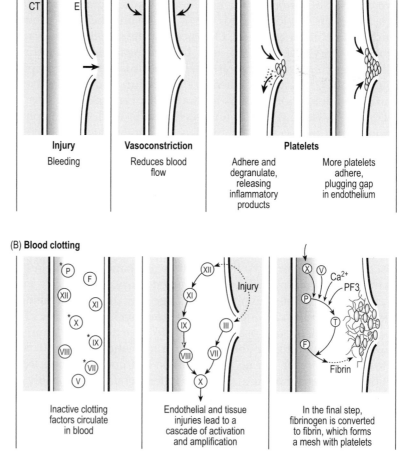

(A) The role of platelets

| **Injury** | **Vasoconstriction** | **Platelets** | |
| Bleeding | Reduces blood flow | Adhere and degranulate, releasing inflammatory products | More platelets adhere, plugging gap in endothelium |

(B) Blood clotting

| Inactive clotting factors circulate in blood | Endothelial and tissue injuries lead to a cascade of activation and amplification | In the final step, fibrinogen is converted to fibrin, which forms a mesh with platelets |

Fig. 2.3 Haemostasis, showing the role of platelets and the clotting system, both of which are required for a firm stable clot. CT: connective tissue; E: endothelium of vessel wall; P: prothrombin; T: thrombin; F: fibrinogen; PF: platelet factor. Molecules marked with an asterisk require vitamin K for their synthesis in the liver.

Healing and repair

We are now in a position to examine the healing of Wendy's stab wound and the non-healing of Mr X's fracture. To take the wound first, we can recognize five main stages (see Fig. 2.4):

- Haemostasis.
- Inflammation.
- Epidermal regrowth.
- Dermal repair.
- Restoration of elasticity.

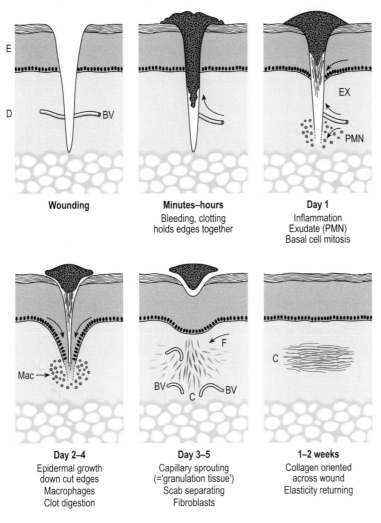

Fig. 2.4 Healing of a clean skin wound, showing the main stages. E: epidermis; D: dermis; BV: blood vessel; EX: exudate; PMN: polymorphs (neutrophils); Mac: macrophages; F: fibroblasts; C: collagen. Note that though healing appears complete at 1–2 weeks, full strength of the scar takes several months to return.

Where there has been extensive loss of tissue, as in burns, repair takes longer and there may in addition be substantial contraction of the wound, with permanent distortion of the tissue. Another rare complication is an excessive overgrowth of collagen and fibrous tissue, for unknown reasons, leading to the formation of bulging unsightly scar tissue known as *keloid*.

A fractured bone is repaired in the same general fashion, with additional special features (see Fig. 2.5). Not only the soft tissues but the bone itself must reunite, and unless great care has been taken to bring the broken ends into precise alignment, a good deal of extra bone has to be first deposited to restore continuity and then remodelled to restore the original shape – which in bad cases may never be fully achieved.

Nerves are a special case. In the central nervous system (brain and spinal cord) nerve cells cannot regenerate and are simply replaced by scar tissue. However, in peripheral nerves individual axons can regrow provided the

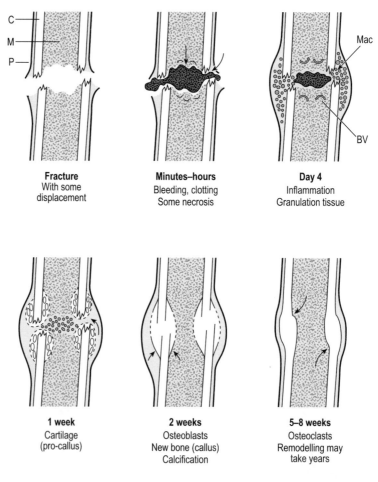

Fracture
With some
displacement

Minutes–hours
Bleeding, clotting
Some necrosis

Day 4
Inflammation
Granulation tissue

1 week
Cartilage
(pro-callus)

2 weeks
Osteoblasts
New bone (callus)
Calcification

5–8 weeks
Osteoclasts
Remodelling may
take years

Fig. 2.5 Healing of a fractured bone, showing the main stages. C: cortex; P: periosteum; M: marrow cavity. Note that strength is restored in a month or two, but if there is bony displacement (as in the example shown here), complete remodelling, under the influence of the surrounding musculature, may take a year or more (all times shown are approximate).

cell body is still alive and there is a tube for them to follow (see Fig. 2.6). This proceeds slowly – about 3 mm per day. Recovery of function may be complete, but in severe injuries fibrous tissue may impede the proper rerouting of the axons, leading to reduced sensory and/or motor function.

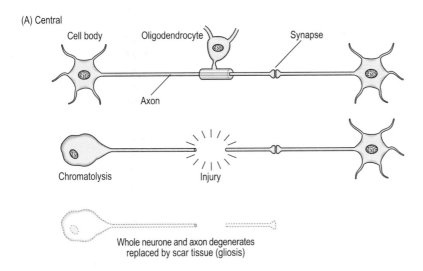

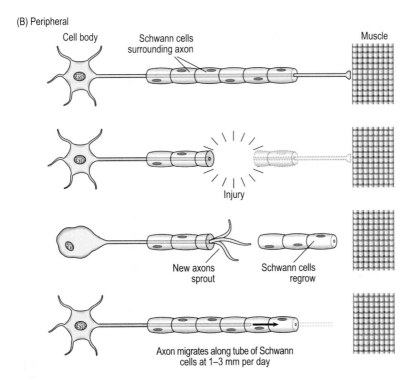

Fig. 2.6 The effect of nerve damage is very different in the central and in the peripheral nervous system.

Impaired healing

Many local factors can interfere with the proper healing of wounds or fractures, the commonest and most important being *infection*. It is practically impossible to prevent contamination of a wound by *staphylococci* from the surrounding skin, and when there has been exposure to soil, as in Mr X's motorcycle accident, *clostridia* such as those that cause tetanus and gas gangrene are also a danger. In addition, healing can be delayed by excessive movement of the affected parts – which is prevented as far as possible by immobilizing them with sutures and/or plaster – while the healing of open wounds can be delayed by the presence of foreign bodies (including sutures!). When the local circulation is deficient, as in legs affected by severe varicose veins, small injuries can lead to chronic non-healing ulcers. Other causes include malnutrition and immune suppression. There are also some general conditions in which healing is impaired (see Table 2.3).

Long-term effects of acute inflammation

There are in essence three major possible outcomes of the inflammatory process:

- Resolution.
- Organization and scarring.
- Death.

In most circumstances, the inflammatory process leads to removal of the offending agent and restoration of the tissues to normal, and this is termed *resolution*. If the tissues damaged cannot regenerate or if the tissue damage has been extensive, *organization* takes place. The ingrowth of capillaries and fibroblasts (called granulation tissue) leads to the production of collagen and a scar is laid down. This will contract to varying degrees to produce some distortion of the tissue. The effect on function may be negligible and cosmetic or it may be dramatic if it affects vital structures such as the brain. Finally, if the offending agent overwhelms the body's defences or the inflammatory response is out of control, the patient may die. This final

Table 2.3 Healing of a wound or fracture can be impaired for many reasons, both local and systemic

1. Local conditions	Comments
Infection	May be secondary to immunodeficiency
Foreign body	
Excessive mobility	Especially fractures
Poor blood supply	e.g. varicose veins
Extensive tissue loss	Causes delay

2. General conditions	Comments
Malnutrition	Especially protein deficiency
Vitamin deficiencies	Especially vitamin C, needed for collagen
Trace metal deficiency	Especially zinc
Diabetes	
Steroid overdosage	Controversial

outcome has become rare with the advent of antibiotics and drugs which modify the inflammatory responses.

Chronic inflammation

The above description has emphasized that acute inflammation is a necessary prelude to healing and repair, and it normally subsides when these processes are complete. Sometimes, however, this does not happen and the inflammation persists for weeks, months, or years – in other words, it becomes *chronic*. There may be an obvious explanation: for example, the original stimulus to inflammation may not have been removed, as happens when foreign material remains in the tissues or in obstinate infections like tuberculosis. Or it may keep on recurring, as with repeated attacks of infection in the same site, e.g. a bone or a kidney. But often there is no evident cause and no acute stage, the inflammation appearing to be of the chronic type from the start, as is seen in many serious diseases, particularly those affecting the joints, lungs, and intestine.

Just as the phagocytic neutrophils were prominent in acute inflammation, in chronic inflammation it is the lymphocytes, plasma cells and macrophages that dominate the response. Chronic inflammation also differs from acute inflammation by the degree of tissue destruction and hence the healing that takes place by organization and scarring. A special type of chronic inflammation is termed *granulomatous*. This is characterized by the formation of a granuloma, which is a collection of macrophages sometimes surrounded by a rim of lymphocytes. Granulomas vary depending on the cause, but some common features are listed in Table 2.4. Often the cause is microbial (e.g. a focus of tubercle or leprosy bacilli), and then *lymphocytes* are also prominent, indicating that the immune system has become involved, as will be described in Chapter 7. This type of granuloma is also

Table 2.4 Granulomas represent foci of macrophage activity and may be due to a variety of causes. Further details of infectious and immunological granulomas will be found in Chapter 7

Causes	Comments
Foreign irritants	
Non-toxic	'Low turnover', e.g. splinters, talc
Toxic	'High turnover', e.g. silica
Infectious organisms	
Resistant to killing	Tuberculosis, leprosy, syphilis, *Histoplasma*, *Cryptococcus*, *Chlamydia* (lymphogranuloma inguinale)
Resistant to digestion	Streptococcal cell walls
In immunodeficiency	e.g. chronic granulomatous disease
Unknown cause	
Sarcoidosis	Lung, liver, spleen, bones
Temporal arteritis	
Wegener's granulomatosis	
Eosinophilic granuloma of bone	

found in a number of serious diseases of unknown cause, of which the commonest are sarcoidosis and Crohn's disease; a microbial origin is naturally suspected but none has ever been proved.

A chronic peptic ulcer is a good example of chronic inflammation and its outcome. The stomach normally produces acid to aid digestion of food. The mucous layer in the stomach protects the mucosa from self-digestion. If for any reason the protective factors are altered, the acid will lead to damage of the gastric mucosa. This sets up an acute inflammatory response as discussed above ('acute gastritis'). If the offending stimulus persists, a balance will be struck between the persistence of injury from the acid and the body's attempt at trying to heal the defect (the ulcer). A number of possible scenarios then result. If the condition is treated with acid-reducing drugs, healing will take place and the ulcer will disappear with only a scar within the wall. Or the ulcer may persist for many years without progressing and a balance is set between continued insult and inflammation/healing. If the acid causes excessive damage, the ulcer may progress and lead to perforation of the gastric wall and the patient may then present with signs of peritonitis (inflammation of the peritoneal cavity). Erosion of the large blood vessels within the mucosa can lead to massive bleeding into the gastrointestinal tract or peritoneal cavity. If the ulcer persists for a long time, excessive scarring may occur as the body tries to hold the offence in check, and this may distort the wall and eventually the cavity of the stomach. If the scarring is circumferential, it will produce an 'hour glass' stomach. If the scarring occurs at the outlet, it will cause obstruction to the flow of food to the small bowel and hence lead to vomiting.

This example illustrates the array of changes and possible outcomes of chronic inflammation. Chronic inflammatory disorders are some of the commonest and most debilitating illnesses encountered in medical practice.

THE TERMINOLOGY OF INFLAMMATION

Generally, the suffix -*itis* added to the name of an organ or tissue denotes that it is inflamed, *acute* or *chronic* being added as appropriate (see Appendix 1 for a complete list). However, one should be cautious about the use of certain terms, which imply more knowledge of the pathology than actually exists. For example, the term *cellulitis* is often applied to a spreading deep-seated infection, but the cells affected are no more or less inflamed that in many other conditions. Similarly, the term *fibrositis*, though widely used to describe chronic localized muscular pain and tenderness, with associated swelling, nodularity, etc., does not correspond to any precise pathology, and indeed is avoided by doctors and pathologists, genuine inflammatory conditions of muscle being referred to as *myositis*. (This does not mean, of course, that the pain and tenderness are imaginary – simply that their pathology is not understood.)

CELL DEATH

Cell death is one possible outcome of the inflammatory response. Death in tissues as a result of inflammation occurs by necrosis. This needs to be distinguished from another type of cell death called apoptosis in which the inflammatory response does not play a role.

Necrosis

Cells dying from most forms of injury undergo a fairly standardized series of changes known as *necrosis*, which include swelling, loss of distinction between nucleus, mitochondria, etc., and the appearance of vacuoles and clumps of chromatin (see Fig. 2.7). Release of enzymes from the dying cell may also damage surrounding cells. At the level of the tissue, necrosis can be classified as coagulative, liquefactive, caseous, fibrinoid and gangrenous (see Table 2.2).

In coagulative necrosis, the tissues are seen to be dead but the ghost outline of the architecture is still visible. Liquefactive refers to tissues taking on the appearance of being liquid-like and occurs characteristically in the brain. Strong hydrolytic enzymes degrade the tissues to produce fluid-like tissue debris. Caseous necrosis is a characteristic feature of tuberculosis and refers to the necrotic tissue taking on the appearance of crumbly cheese. The term fibrinoid is used when the necrotic tissue resembles fibrin. Gangrene is not really a specific type of necrosis but is the term given to describe black dead tissues.

Apoptosis

Unlike necrosis, this is a purposeful type of cell death. Many cells die in the course of normal development and tissue modelling, the formation of separate fingers from the embryonic flipper-like hand being a familiar example. Here a quite different process is used to get rid of the unwanted cells, known as *apoptosis* or by the more descriptive name 'programmed cell death'. The cell is literally dismantled in a tidy fashion, with no damage to its neighbours. Hence, unlike necrosis where there is usually an inflammatory component, no inflammatory cells are seen during death due to apoptosis. Another very characteristic change is the cutting of the DNA into pieces of standard length by enzymes, which can readily be seen when the DNA is run on a gel (Fig. 2.7).

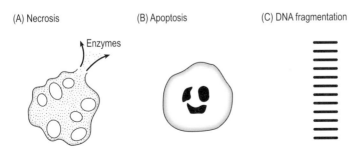

(A) Necrosis   (B) Apoptosis   (C) DNA fragmentation

Enzymes

Fig. 2.7 Two kinds of cell death: In necrosis (A) the cells become vacuolated, swell, and break open releasing their contents (enzymes, etc.), which may damage surrounding tissues and lead to inflammation. In apoptosis (B) – programmed cell death – there is a characteristic fragmentation of the nucleus and the DNA is cut by enzymes into uniform lengths (C).

Tutorial 2

Test your understanding of tissue injury and repair by planning answers to the following essay questions. Remember that in an exam you are not expected to regurgitate every single relevant fact, but to show that you understand the problem, know *most* of the facts, and can think about them intelligently.

QUESTIONS

1. Name three types of cell and three types of molecule involved in acute inflammation.

2. List, in order of probability, the factors that might prevent a fractured bone healing.

3. Why and how does blood clot?

4. What do you understand by 'chronic inflammation'? Give three examples.

5. We would be better off without pain. Discuss.

6. Cell death after injury: murder or suicide?

ANSWERS

1. Mast cells, neutrophils, vascular endothelial cells, lymphocytes; histamine, arachidonic acid, prostaglandins, leukotrienes, Hageman factor, complement, cytokines, acute phase proteins. You will read more about complement and lymphocytes in Chapter 5, but all the others have been mentioned in this chapter.

2. Infection, foreign body, movement, general disease (see Table 2.4 for a list). Movement of the two parts is a most effective way to prevent healing, but it is of course usually avoided by immobilization.

3. The purpose of blood clotting is to prevent loss of blood following damage to a blood vessel; in all other circumstances it is highly undesirable. It occurs by a series of activation steps involving at least 12 serum- or tissue-derived molecules, culminating in the formation of fibrin. The fibrinolytic pathway normally prevents the clot spreading to form a thrombus (see Chapter 8 for details of unwanted and abnormal clotting).

4. Chronic inflammation implies a time course lasting more than a few days, but it also implies a major involvement of macrophages. Normally the two go together, the macrophages collecting at the site of inflammation to help dispose of microbes or foreign bodies that cannot be dealt with by the neutrophils, etc., of the acute inflammatory response. Sometimes, however, there is no obvious acute stage, and a chronic inflammatory lesion appears 'from nowhere'.

5. Pain is clearly useful when it instructs the body to rest an affected part (e.g. the heart following a heart attack) or to avoid a dangerous stimulus. Patients who do not feel pain in the hands or feet (e.g. sufferers from diabetic neuropathy or diseases of the nervous system such as syringomyelia) can inflict severe injuries on themselves without noticing. But the chronic pain of, for example, some cancers serves no useful purpose and any effective treatment is justified.

6. Cell death after injury could be either 'murder' (necrosis) or 'suicide' (apoptosis), depending on the type of injury. If you burn yourself, cell and tissue death will occur owing to both direct injury to cells and injury secondary to ischaemia caused by damage to blood vessels. Subsequent infection due to breach of the skin barrier will contribute further to necrosis. All these changes represent an *inflammatory* response to the injury. In contrast, injury due to radiation may be more subtle. A brief exposure may only induce damage to a small segment of DNA within the nucleus. Cells have mechanisms for dealing with such damage, since some degree of DNA repair is required constantly. But if the cell is unable to repair the damage, it also has the ability to set into operation a programme for cell suicide – apoptosis, or 'programmed cell death'. However, if the suicide-inducing genes are themselves damaged, the cell may be able to survive and replicate, producing daughter cells with the genetic damage. This may be the first step in the production of tumours (see Chapter 12 for more on this). You should be able to think of other examples of necrosis and apoptosis.

FURTHER READING

Here are some longer pathology textbooks which cover the subject in more detail:

Cotran R S, Kumar V, Robbins S L 1994 Pathologic basis of disease, 5th edn. Saunders, Philadelphia, 1400 pp
A large and beautifully written American textbook, with a good chapter on genetic disorders.

Govan A D T, Macfarlane P S, Callander R 1995 Pathology illustrated, 4th edn. Churchill Livingstone, Edinburgh, 843 pp

Stevens A, Lowe J 1995 Pathology, Mosby, London, 535 pp
With copious colour illustrations and accompanying slide atlas.

Vardaxis N J 1995 Pathology for the health sciences. Churchill Livingstone, Edinburgh, 827 pp
Written for (Australian) health science students, this substantial book covers essentially the same ground as Muir, etc., though with more self-test and case-study material than most.

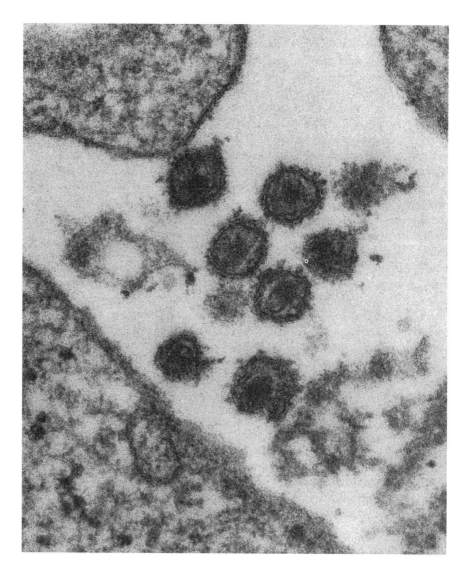

Human immunodeficiency virus (HIV) budding from an infected cell. HIV is one of the most recent additions to the infectious organisms that afflict man, which range from the tiny viruses, only visible (as here) in the electron microscope, through the microscopic bacteria, fungi, and protozoa, to the large multicellular worms. In this chapter we consider the infectious organisms of medical importance.

(Reproduced with kind permission from: Madeley C R & Field A M 1988 Virus Morphology, 2nd edn. Churchill Livingstone, Edinburgh)

Infectious organisms

■ CONTENTS

Case 3.1

Dr Petrie returned from a holiday in India in good health, but within a week he was suffering from high evening temperature, muscle pains, and general weakness, with a slight cough and headache. Since he had taken a course of antimalarials, he treated himself for influenza, but the condition did not improve. His own GP, suspecting typhoid fever, referred him to a tropical disease centre, where a thick blood film showed the presence of *Plasmodium falciparum*, the parasite of malignant tertian malaria. Oral treatment with quinine and mefloquine allowed an uneventful recovery.

Infectious disease is still a major cause of illness in the tropics and, with today's emphasis on travel, in temperate countries too (Table 3.1). Dr Petrie was unlucky in that his malaria was resistant to his chosen antimalarial

Table 3.1 Infectious diseases were responsible for approximately 17 000 000 deaths in 1995, predominantly in tropical countries (WHO figures)

Disease	Mortality
Acute respiratory infection	4 400 000
Diarrhoeal diseases	3 100 000
Tuberculosis	3 100 000
Malaria	2 100 000
Hepatitis B	1 100 000
AIDS	1 000 000
Measles	1 000 000
Neonatal tetanus	500 000
Whooping cough	355 000
Roundworms	165 000

(probably chloroquine) and that it did not show the 'textbook' pattern of a 2- or 3-day fever cycle. He was lucky in having a GP not content to put his symptoms down to 'flu', and in the availability of experts in tropical diseases. However, his symptoms *could* have been due to influenza (a viral infection) or typhoid (a bacterial infection), as well as many other exotic conditions. The message is, therefore, that you need to know something about infectious organisms of all types, the diseases they cause (these will be described in Chapter 4) and how they are prevented and treated (see Chapter 8). In this chapter, we will take a look at the organisms themselves.

The one thing all infectious organisms have in common is that they are *parasites* of a larger host (e.g. man). Otherwise, they differ widely, from the tiny viruses and prions, only visible in the electron microscope, to worms and insects clearly visible to the naked eye. Table 3.2 and Figure 3.1 list some of the important distinguishing features of the main classes of organism, together with some of the not always very logical terminology used to classify them.

Table 3.2 The major classes of infectious organism and their principal distinguishing features

Class	Visibility	Structure	Typical diseases
Prions	Electron microscope	Protein	BSE (in cattle), scrapie (in sheep), kuru, CJD (in man)
Viruses	Electron microscope	DNA or RNA plus protein	Influenza, polio, AIDS, measles, mumps, colds
Bacteria	Light microscope	Single-cell (procaryotic)[1]	'Strep throat', TB, tetanus, 'staph' abscess, syphilis
Protozoa	Light microscope	Single-cell (eucaryotic)[1]	Malaria, leishmaniasis, giardiasis, amoebiasis
Fungi	Light microscope Naked eye (some)	Single-cell or multicellular	Candidiasis ('thrush'), ringworm
Worms	Naked eye	Multicellular	Schistosomiasis, hookworm, tapeworm
Insects	Naked eye	(Ectoparasites)[2]	Head/body lice, scabies

[1] For a definition of procaryotic and eucaryotic cell structure, see text.
[2] Inhabiting the skin only. The term microbe is sometimes loosely applied to bacteria, microorganism to bacteria, protozoa, and small fungi, and parasite to protozoa and worms, but infectious organism is a better term for all of these. Note that the vast majority of bacteria, fungi, protozoa, and worms are not parasitic but free-living.

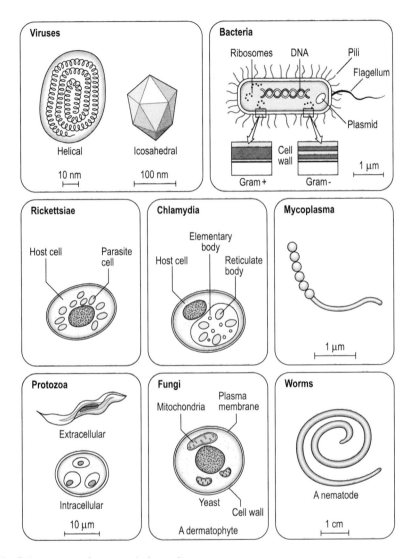

Fig. 3.1 Structure of some typical parasites.

VIRUSES AND PRIONS

Viruses

Viruses are not so much living organisms as sets of instructions for their own reproduction, relying on a host cell to provide the translating machinery (thus the concept of a 'computer virus' is not so far-fetched). Their instructions are in the form of either DNA or RNA, either being sufficient to code for the various enzymes and other proteins that make up the complete virus particle.

Viruses exhibit a remarkable regularity of structure, based on the way their outer proteins or *capsids* are packed, which may be (1) helical, with capsids projecting from a spiral of RNA or (2) icosahedral, with 20 triangular faces and a fixed number of capsids, e.g. 252 for adenoviruses. In addition, those viruses which spread by budding (see below) are surrounded by a lipid envelope derived from the host cell. Viruses are generally classified on the basis of these properties, as Table 3.3 shows. Note that most DNA viruses are double-stranded, while many RNA viruses are single-stranded (and helical).

Entering, leaving, and damaging the host cell

Since viruses depend on host cells for replication, they are obligate intracellular parasites, which means they need a mechanism for entering and leaving cells. Entry is by attachment to particular molecules on the surface of the host cell, which are referred to as *receptors* for the virus in question,

Table 3.3 The principal viruses of medical importance

Nucleic acid	Enveloped	Non-enveloped
DNA (double-stranded)	Herpes viruses HSV 1, HSV 2, VZV, EBV, CMV	Adenoviruses (common colds)
	Pox viruses Variola (smallpox), vaccinia (cowpox), molluscum contagiosum	Papovaviruses Papilloma (warts)
	Hepadna viruses Hepatitis B	Parvovirus (single-stranded)
RNA (single-stranded)	Orthomyxovirus Influenza A, B, C	Picorna virus Rhinovirus, enterovirus,
	Paramyxovirus Measles, mumps, RSV, parainfluenza	polio, Coxsackie, hepatitis A, echovirus
	Coronavirus (colds)	
	Rhabdovirus Rabies	
	Arenavirus/filovirus Lassa, Marburg, Ebola	
	Togavirus Rubella	
	Flavivirus Yellow fever, dengue, hepatitis C	
	Retrovirus HIV 1,2; HTLV 1,2	Reovirus (double-stranded) Rotavirus (double-stranded)

though their normal function is something quite different. For example, HIV attaches to a molecule known as CD4, and, because this is found mainly on T lymphocytes and to some extent on macrophages, these are the cells predominantly infected. In the same way, the Epstein-Barr virus (EBV) attaches to a molecule whose normal role is to bind complement to B lymphocytes (see Chapter 5 for what T and B lymphocytes and complement are).

Exit from cells is either by rupturing (*lysing*) the host cell, in which case it will die, or by budding off from the cell surface, surrounded by an envelope of host membrane (see plate on page 32), which may leave the cell intact, unless the virus has already disrupted the nucleus, as DNA viruses usually do. Note that an enveloped virus must insert a suitable molecule into the envelope to allow it to attach to a receptor on the next host cell; the well-known Gp 120 and CD4 molecules play these roles in HIV infection.

Lysis and nuclear disruption are two ways in which viruses can damage the host cell and cause disease, but other outcomes are also possible. Viruses may persist even after apparent recovery, causing the patient to be a *carrier* (e.g. hepatitis B); they may remain *latent*, as herpes viruses do in the central nervous system, to flare up many years later (e.g. shingles after chickenpox); or they may *transform* the host cell into one that divides continuously – in other words a tumour. Transformation is usually due to the possession by the virus of an *oncogene* (i.e. tumour-inducing gene) which closely resembles a normal host gene whose function is to stimulate cell division. For further details on oncogenes and tumours, see Chapters 1 and 12.

The ways in which viruses can be eliminated by the immune system, and their ingenious strategies for resisting elimination, are discussed in Chapter 6, and you will come across them again when we discuss vaccination – the most effective method yet devised to control virus infection (Chapter 8).

Prions

For many years it was assumed that an infectious organism must contain at least some nucleic acid – otherwise how could it replicate? But long and detailed study of a group of food-transmitted diseases known as the *spongiform encephalopathies* seems to have established that they can be transmitted by small protein molecules, which have been baptized *prions* (see Table 3.2). One theory is that these act as templates for host-derived proteins to clump together in the brain, rather in the way that crystals form. Another theory is that 'normal' prions must be altered and accumulate to become pathogenic. The 'British beef' scare was based on the idea that they may spread from one species to another, which is unfortunately going to take many years to absolutely prove or disprove.

BACTERIA

Bacteria are single-celled organisms, the vast majority of which are capable of fully independent existence, being found in soil and water, often under conditions of temperature, pressure, background radiation, etc., that would be totally inhospitable to higher forms of life. A few species of bacteria have adopted a parasitic lifestyle, colonizing the body surface and intestines of higher animals, where they do no harm and may even be useful. Unfortunately a small number of these can enter and damage the tissues of the host, leading to bacterial disease and sometimes death. The science of *microbiology* originally developed when the link between these microscopic creatures and diseases such as tuberculosis, anthrax, and cholera was established in the late 1800s by Pasteur, Koch, and others.

The bacterial cell is unique in having a cell wall and lacking a nucleus; this type of cell is called *procaryotic* in contrast to the *eucaryotic* structure found in all higher animals from protozoa to mammals (Fig. 3.1). This difference is not just academic; it helps to explain why immunity, vaccination, and antibiotics are generally more effective against bacteria than against parasitic protozoa, fungi and worms. More about this in Chapters 6 and 8. Outside the cell wall, bacteria may have *capsules* (to protect them against phagocytes), *flagella* (for motility) or *pili* (for attachment to mucous surfaces).

Unlike viruses, bacteria are not always named after the disease they cause, but classified into groups according to (1) shape and (2) the nature of their cell wall (Table 3.4). Round bacteria are called *cocci*, rod-shaped ones *bacilli*. Those with thick cell walls that stain blue with iodine and do not decolorize with alcohol are called *Gram-positive*; if they do decolorize they are *Gram-negative*. The Gram stain is one of the most useful rapid diagnostic tests, and can be performed in a few minutes, whereas most other tests require the bacteria to be cultured on special agar-based plates at 37°C overnight or longer, so as to multiply and give rise to *colonies*, whose shape and colour often help in identification. It is possible that all bacterial typing will eventually be done by detecting surface antigenic differences with *monoclonal antibodies* (see Chapter 5), but at present antibodies are mainly used for the precise identification of subtypes or for distinguishing otherwise very similar species of bacteria.

Intracellular and extracellular bacteria

As mentioned above, most bacteria are free-living. Some can be free-living or parasitic (the tetanus bacillus is an example). But even among the parasitic ones, some are 'more parasitic' than others, being able to live inside the cells of the host, rather as viruses do. Note however that they are *not* dependent on the host cell for their replication, and most of them can be cultured in the laboratory in the absence of any host material. Others prefer to remain in the extracellular spaces – tissue fluid, mucous surfaces, blood etc. The significance of intracellular versus extracellular existence will be appreciated when we consider how the immune system tries to eliminate bacteria (Chapter 6).

Atypical bacteria

Not all bacteria conform precisely to the above description (see Table 3.4, bottom). Some have an unusual spiral shape, including the organism that causes syphilis. Others (the Rickettsiae and Chlamydiae) need to be inside

Table 3.4 The principal bacteria of medical importance

Gram stain	Cocci	Bacilli

Positive	Staphylococci
	Streptococci
		Anthrax bacillus
		Clostridia
		    C. tetani (tetanus)[1]
		    C. perfringens (gas gangrene)
		    C. botulinum
		Corynebacteria (diphtheria)
		Listeria

Negative	Neisseria
	    Meningococcus
	    Gonococcus
		Salmonella
		Shigella (enteritis)
		Escherichia
		Yersinia (plague)
		Pseudomonas
		Proteus
		Vibrio (cholera)
		Haemophilus
		Helicobacter (gastritis)
		Brucella
		Bordetella (whooping cough)
		Legionella

Gram stain not used		Mycobacteria (TB, leprosy)

Atypical structure
  Spiral
	Spirochaetes
	    Treponema (syphilis)
	    Borrelia (Lyme disease)
	    Leptospira	

Obligate intracellular	Rickettsiae (typhus) Chlamydiae (trachoma, psittacosis)	
No cell wall	Mycoplasma	

[1]*Where a bacterium causes a specific disease which cannot be deduced from its name, this is shown in parentheses.*

host cells in order to replicate, as viruses do, while the Mycoplasmas are even more virus-like in lacking cell walls altogether. Some Gram-positive bacilli (anthrax, clostridia) are able to survive for long periods by forming *spores*.

Bacterial disease

In Chapter 4 we shall consider the various ways in which infectious organisms cause disease. Here we will just mention that many of the harmful effects of bacteria are due to the secretion of *toxins*; tetanus, diphtheria, and cholera are well-known examples. But as with all types of infectious organism, damage can also be caused by the immune system reacting against the bacteria. This is called *immunopathology*, and will be further explained in Chapter 7.

PROTOZOA

These are also single-celled organisms, but their cells are *eucaryotic*, which makes them much closer to the cells of higher animals in structure and function (see Fig. 3.1), and correspondingly more difficult for the immune system, or drugs, to eliminate. Though some protozoal diseases occur all over the world, the majority of the really unpleasant ones are confined to the tropics, usually because they are transmitted by insect vectors that are only found there. An excellent example is *malaria*, which was widespread in Europe until public health measures eliminated the mosquito breeding grounds, but is still – increasingly – a problem in tropical countries, as Dr Petrie learned to his cost. Table 3.5 lists the protozoa of medical importance.

FUNGI

Fungi come in an enormous range of shapes and sizes, and only a handful are of medical importance as parasites (Table 3.6). These include some that inhabit the skin, hair, or nails, and others that colonize mucous membranes – *Candida albicans* (thrush) being the best known of these. There are also some potentially very dangerous fungi that can colonize internal organs,

Table 3.5 The principal protozoa of medical importance

Habitat in host	Means of spread	
	Insects	Water, food, etc.
Extracellular	African trypanosome (free in blood)	*Amoeba* *Giardia* (intestine) *Cryptosporidium* *Trichomonas* (urogenital)
Intracellular	Malaria (liver: red cell) *Leishmania* (macrophage) S. American trypanosome	*Toxoplasma* (macrophage)

Table 3.6 The principal fungi of medical importance

Affecting skin, hair, nails	May invade soft tissue	Normally in lungs	May invade lungs, brain, other organs
Trichophyton *Epidermophyton* *Microsporum*	*Sporothrix* *Candida* *Actinomyces*[2]	*Pneumocystis*[1]	Aspergillus *Blastomyces* Coccidioides *Cryptococcus* *Histoplasma* *Candida*

[1] *Pneumocystis was formerly classified as a protozoan.*
[2] *Though resembling a fungus, Actinomyces is now classified as a bacterium.*

especially the lung. Like protozoa, they are difficult to eliminate because of their eucaryotic cell structure and, in some cases, the possession of tough cellulose or chitin outer cell walls. Fungal infections are becoming increasingly important as *opportunists* – that is, organisms that cause disease only in patients with deficient immune systems (see below).

WORMS

Worms (or *helminths*) are, like protozoa, a minor cause of disease in temperate areas but a major one in the tropics. This similarity, plus the fact that the immune system is almost powerless against either of them, is probably why the study of protozoa and worms is traditionally but illogically lumped together as *parasitology*, in fact they are no more or less parasites than the measles virus or a staphylococcus. Worms are large multicellular animals, visible to the naked eye and sometimes several inches or even feet long; thus they are certainly not *microorganisms*. Only a few are important human pathogens, but these include some extremely chronic and destructive ones (Table 3.7).

INSECTS AND OTHER VECTORS

Most people are familiar with lice, mites and fleas as a cause of itching skin rashes; because they affect the outside of the body, these are referred to as *ectoparasites* (Table 3.8). Insects also play an important role as *vectors* for other infectious organisms, and so do some larger animals such as snails.

Table 3.7 The principal worms of medical importance

	Means of spread	
	Insect or other vector	**Water, food, etc.**
Roundworms (nematodes)	*Onchocerca* (fly) *Wuchereria* (mosquito) *Loa loa* (fly)	*Ascaris* Hookworm *Toxocara* *Trichinella* *Strongyloides*
Tapeworms (cestodes)		*Taenia solium* (pork) *Taenia saginata* (beef) *Diphyllobothrium* *Hymenolepis* *Echinococcus* ('hydatid')
Flukes (trematodes)	Schistosomes (snail) *Schistosoma mansoni* *S. haematobium* *S. japonicum* *Clonorchis* *Paragonimus*	

Table 3.8 Ectoparasites of medical importance

Mites	*Sarcoptes* (scabies)
Lice	*Pediculus* (head, body) *Phthirus* (pubic)
Fleas	*Tunga* (tropics only)
Bugs	*Cimex* (bedbug)

Note: Other biting insects are important as disease vectors; see Table 3.9.

In such cases, the alternative host (mosquito, snail) is an essential part of the parasite life-cycle (Table 3.9). There are also infections which can be accidentally acquired by man from their normal animal host; these are known as *zoonoses* and include some of the most dangerous and rapidly fatal infections of all (Table 3.10).

Table 3.9 Transmission of disease by insects and other animals

Type of organism	Disease	Vector
Viruses	Yellow fever	Mosquito (from man or monkeys)
	Dengue	Mosquito
Rickettsiae	Typhus	Body lice, mites, ticks
Bacteria	Plague	Fleas (from rats)
	Relapsing fever	Ticks (from man or rodents)
	Lyme disease	Ticks (from mice, deer)
	Bartonella	Sandflies
Protozoa	Malaria	Mosquito
	Babesiosis	Ticks (from cattle)
	Sleeping sickness (African trypanosomiasis)	Tsetse fly
	Chagas' disease (S. American trypanosomiasis)	Reduviid bugs
	Leishmaniasis	Sandflies (from man or dog)
Worms	Elephantiasis (*W. bancrofti*)	Mosquito
	Dipetalonema	Flies
	Loaiasis (*Loa loa*)	Flies
	Onchocerciasis	Simulium flies
	Schistosomiasis	Snails
	Fascioliasis	Snails
	Paragonimiasis	Snails

Table 3.10 Some important disease acquired from animals (zoonoses)

Type of organism	Disease	Animal host	How acquired
Viruses	Lassa fever	Bush rat	Urine, blood
	Marburg fever	Monkeys (?)	
	Ebola fever		
	Rabies	Dog, fox, etc.	Bite
Rickettsiae	Q fever	Cattle	Inhalation
Chlamydiae	Psittacosis	Birds	Inhalation
Bacteria	Anthrax	Cattle, etc.	Contact, inhalation
	Plague	Rats	Flea bite
	Brucellosis	Cow, goat, pig	Contact, milk
	Salmonella	Dairy, poultry	Food
	Leptospirosis	Rat	Food
	Tuberculosis	Cattle, birds	Inhalation
Protozoa	Toxoplasmosis	Cat	Faecal–oral
	Cryptosporidiosis	Mammals, birds	Faecal–oral
	Leishmaniasis	Rodents, dog	Insect bite
	S. American trypanosomiasis	Pets, armadillo	Insect bite
Fungi	Cryptococcosis	Birds	Inhalation
	Histoplasmosis	Birds, bats,	Inhalation
Worms	*Taenia* (tapeworm)	Cattle, pigs	Faecal–oral
	Toxocara	Dogs, cats	Faecal–oral
	Echinococcus	Dog	Faecal–oral
	Trichinella	Rat, pig	Faecal–oral
	Strongyloides	(Dog)	Skin

OPPORTUNISTIC INFECTIONS

As already mentioned, some organisms only cause disease in patients with deficient immune systems (see Chapter 7 for details of immunodeficiency), and these are increasingly important for three reasons. Firstly, more children with congenital immunodeficiencies survive nowadays because of better diagnosis and treatment. Secondly, most transplant patients need to be treated with immunosuppressive drugs, sometimes for life. And thirdly there is the effect of the AIDS epidemic, which threatens millions of people with prolonged and progressive immunodeficiency. The result is that a group of previously minor or even unknown organisms has become medically important; a good example is the fungus *Pneumocystis carinii*, a harmless commensal of the normal lung, which hardly featured in microbiology textbooks until the first cases of AIDS started dying of pneumocystis pneumonia. Table 3.11 lists some other opportunists.

Table 3.11 Some important opportunistic infections

Type of organism	Disease/ organism	Effect in healthy individual	Effect in immunodeficient patient
Viruses	Herpes		
	simplex[1]	Vesicular rash	Reactivation
	VZV[1]	Chickenpox	Severe shingles
	CMV[1]	Mild or none	Lung, brain, eye
	EBV	Glandular fever	Burkitt's lymphoma
	Measles		Severe measles
	(attenuated vaccine)		
Bacteria	*Strep. pneumoniae*		Repeated pneumonia
	Staph. aureus	Local	Disseminated
	Pseudomonas	None	Pneumonia
	Mycobacteria[1]	None	Disseminated TB
	Nocardia[1]	None	Lung, brain, skin
	Listeria[1]		Brain
Protozoa	*Toxoplasma*[1]	None	Brain, eye
	Cryptosporidium[1]	Diarrhoea	Weight loss
	Babesia	None	Malaria-like
	Isospora[1]	Mild diarrhoea	Chronic diarrhoea
Fungi	*Candida*[1]	Thrush	Disseminated
	Pneumocystis[1]	None	Pneumonia
	Cryptococcus[1]	Rare	Meningitis
	Histoplasma[1]	Pneumonia	Disseminated
	Aspergillus	Lung	Brain, heart
Worms	*Strongyloides*[1]	None	Systemic spread

[1] *These opportunists are particularly common in AIDS patients.*

FURTHER READING

There are many excellent large textbooks devoted to infectious organisms, differing mainly in whether they include all or only some of the classes of 'parasite'.

Brock T D, Madigan M T 1988 Biology of microorganisms, 5th edn. Prentice-Hall International, Englewood Cliffs, N J, 833 pp.
Viruses, bacteria, fungi, protozoa.

Cox F E G (ed) 1993 Modern parasitology, 2nd edn. Blackwell Scientific, Oxford, 276 pp
Protozoa, worms, insects.

Muller R, Baker J R 1990 Medical parasitology. Lippincott, Philadelphia, 168 pp
Protozoa, worms, insects.

Sleigh J D, Timbury M C 1986 Notes on medical bacteriology, 2nd edn. Churchill Livingstone, Edinburgh, 403 pp

Timbury M C 1983 Notes on medical virology, 7th edn. Churchill Livingstone, Edinburgh, 155 pp

Topley and Wilson's principles of bacteriology, virology, and immunity, 8th edn. 1990. Arnold, London, 2736 pp
Viruses, bacteria.

Tutorial 3

Here are some microbiological topics that frequently crop up in exams. You could usefully imagine having to write either a 10-minute short answer or a 30-minute essay.

QUESTIONS

1. When speaking of viruses, what is meant by (1) single-stranded, (2) icosahedral, (3) enveloped?

2. What can be learned by examining bacteria with a microscope?

3. Name three protozoal infections, as contrasted as possible.

4. Some fungi are important opportunists. Explain and discuss this statement.

5. How do the cells of worms differ from those of (1) bacteria, (2) protozoa?

6. Discuss the role of insects in disease.

ANSWERS

1. 'Single'- and 'double-stranded' refer to the configuration of the DNA or RNA making up the viral genome. 'Icosahedral' describes the 20-faceted shape of many DNA and RNA viruses, contrasting with the helical structure of some RNA viruses. 'Enveloped' means surrounded by a host cell-derived lipid membrane, budded off from the host cell.

2. In stained preparations, spherical *cocci* can easily be distinguished from rod-shaped *bacilli*, curved *vibrios*, or corkscrew-shaped *spirochaetes*. The spores of e.g. clostridia would also be visible. The Gram stain will further distinguish positive (purple) from negative (pink) bacteria (see Table 3.4 for the value of this). Mycobacteria can be identified by the Ziehl-Neelsen stain, which depends on resistance to both acid and alcohol. Immunofluorescent staining with suitable antibodies can be used to identify surface antigens with great precision.

3. Amoeba (water-borne, extracellular); malaria (mosquito-borne, intracellular); *Toxoplasma* (intracellular, opportunistic, zoonosis); *Leishmania* (intracellular, insect-borne, zoonosis); African trypanosome (free in blood).

4. An opportunist is an infectious organism causing mild or no disease in healthy people but serious disease when immunity is suppressed or deficient. Several fungi fall into this category, notably *Candida*, *Pneumocystis*, *Toxoplasma*, *Cryptococcus*. The assumption is that a normal immune system can keep these infections in check, though we do not always know exactly how. Fungal infections are becoming increasingly important because of the number of immunodeficient individuals in the population.

5. Worms are multicellular (metazoan) organisms, made up of *eucaryotic* cells, very similar to those of the mammals, fish, birds, etc, they often parasitize. Protozoa are also eucaryotes, but *single-celled* (or, as some parasitologists would say, acellular). Bacteria are single-celled *procaryotes*, with a radically different cell structure (see Fig. 3.1). Don't confuse procaryotes with protozoa!

6. Their major importance is as *vectors*, essential for the transmission of many serious infections, especially in the tropics. Look back at Table 3.9 for a list of these. Huge efforts are being made to eradicate mosquitoes in particular, since they can transmit malaria, elephantiasis, and yellow fever, to name but a few. A less important, though irritating, role is as parasites of the skin – lice, mites, bugs, and fleas.

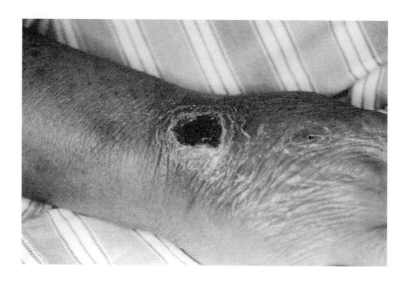

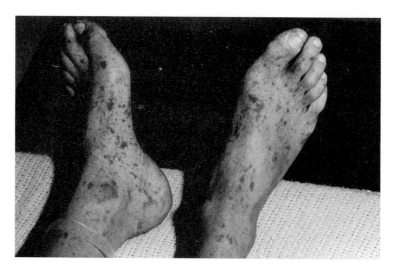

Two life-threatening conditions with easily visible skin changes.
Top: *this intravenous drip site has become contaminated with*
Staphylococcus aureus, probably from the nose of the doctor who
set it up. ***Bottom:*** *the rash of meningococcal septicaemia. Both of*
these conditions are due to bacterial toxins, but the pathology is
quite different. In this chapter we discuss toxins and other ways in
which infectious organisms can cause disease.

(Reproduced with kind permission from Dr Geoffrey M. S. Scott, Dept of Clinical Microbiology, UCL Hospitals NHS Trust, London.)

Infectious disease

4

During World War I (1914–18), over 2 million British troops were wounded, and of these some 2400 developed tetanus – an average rate of 1.2 per thousand casualties, with 34% deaths. However, during the first 3 months (August–October 1914) this ratio was 6.7 per thousand, of which about 85% died. Meanwhile the rate among civilians was only about 1 per million. By contrast, after the war was over (1918–19) an epidemic of influenza swept through Europe, causing about 20 000 000 deaths, in soldiers and civilians alike – far more than the casualties of the entire war.

What can we learn from these terrible figures? Firstly, that some infections are more or less confined to select populations (e.g. tetanus in the wounded), while others can strike anyone (e.g. influenza). Secondly, that the incidence and mortality of some diseases can be drastically affected by treatment. The reduction in tetanus was due to the availability from October 1914 of *antitoxin* – a serum preparation containing antibodies against the toxin that causes all the symptoms – which by World War II (1939–45) had been replaced by the now universal *vaccine*, resulting in a rate of only 0.06 per thousand casualties. The treatment of influenza, on the other hand, has hardly changed since 1920, though a moderately effective vaccine is available for those particularly at risk. The reader can no doubt think of many other infectious diseases that differ in incidence, contagiousness, severity, duration, mortality, and treatability. In this chapter we shall discuss some of the reasons for these differences.

VIRULENCE AND VIRULENCE FACTORS

Surprising as it may seem, the great majority of microorganisms do not behave as if they 'wanted' to make us ill. Indeed, to kill your host is rather like booking into a hotel and immediately blowing it up, with yourself inside! Sometimes the symptoms of disease do make good sense; for example, damage to respiratory epithelium resulting in the induction of copious mucus and sneezing is an excellent way for the influenza virus to spread to other hosts; if everyone wore masks, the virus would have great difficulty surviving. Likewise, the induction of diarrhoea helps the spread of intestinal viruses, bacteria, and protozoa. But in the case of the tetanus bacillus, which normally lives in the soil, the infection and death of an occasional human is an accidental event of no significance, since the soil will continue to teem with bacilli and spores. The tendency of an organism to cause disease, whether logical or not, is known as *virulence*, and anything which promotes this is called a *virulence factor*. As Table 4.1 shows, virulence factors can range from fundamental properties of the organism (e.g. the

Table 4.1 The main factors determining the virulence of infectious organisms

Mechanism	Example
Entry	
Attachment to host receptor molecules	Viruses, some bacteria
Destruction of host tissues	
Direct cytopathic effects[1]	Many viruses,
Enzymes	streptococci
Exotoxins[2]	Tetanus, cholera
Multiplication	All except worms
Spread	
Induction of coughing, sneezing	Respiratory viruses
Induction of diarrhoea	Intestinal viruses and bacteria
Location in/on skin	Staphylococci
Animal reservoir	Zoonoses[3]
Escape from host defences[4]	
Inhibition of external defences	*B. pertussis*
Avoidance of phagocytosis	*Strep. pneumoniae*
Destruction of phagocytes	*Staph. aureus*
Avoidance of complement	*Leishmania*
Sequestration	Slow viruses
Antigenic variation	Influenza
Inhibition of lymphocyte function	HIV
Induction of immunopathology[5]	Tuberculosis

[1] *See Table 4.2.*
[2] *See Table 4.3.*
[3] *See Table 3.10.*
[4] *See Chapter 6.*
[5] *See Chapter 7.*

production of tetanus toxin) to subtle strategies for evading host defences, such as the remarkable ability of the influenza virus to vary its surface proteins and confuse the immune system.

What causes disease?

Tetanus and influenza represent the two main ways in which an infectious organism can directly cause disease: the production of *toxins* (nearly always by bacteria) and *cytopathic* effects due to the invasion and destruction of cells (mostly by viruses). However, many organisms neither produce toxins nor invade cells, yet they can cause severe disease or death. Frequently this is an indirect effect, secondary to stimulation of the immune system. This type of disease is called *immunopathology*, and will be dealt with after we have looked at how the immune system normally works (Chapters 5, 6). Here we will discuss the direct causes of disease in more detail.

CYTOPATHIC INFECTIONS

As described in Chapter 3, some viruses rupture cells in exiting from them, and clearly, if this happens on a large scale, there will be considerable tissue destruction. Influenza and the viruses of the common cold in the respiratory tract are typical examples. Other viruses inhibit cell functions, such as protein synthesis; polio in the CNS is an example. Rarely they stimulate cells to grow into a tumour (e.g. carcinoma of the liver following hepatitis B). The microscopically visible changes in infected cells are fairly non-specific: oedema, or 'cloudy swelling', various 'inclusion bodies', 'rounding up', and the fusion of cells into *syncytia* are all signs of virus infection, but are not usually sufficient to pinpoint the precise virus. Table 4.2 lists some of the viruses that do, or do not, cause direct damage to cells. It also includes a few non-viral organisms that damage tissues directly.

Table 4.2 Tissue damage by viruses and other organisms

Mechanism	Examples
Cell lysis	Most respiratory viruses (mucosal cells) Malaria (red cell) HIV (T lymphocytes)
Protein synthesis inhibited	Polio (neurones)
Induction of immunopathology	Tuberculosis
Induction of tumours	Hepatitis B, EB virus, papillomavirus
Physical/mechanical effects	*Ascaris*, hydatid cyst
Persistence without cell lysis	Hepatitis B (liver cell) HIV (monocytes) Herpes viruses (CNS)

TOXINS

The toxins of tetanus and other bacteria are fascinating molecules, because they act in such an amazing variety of ways, the understanding of which requires a good knowledge of cell biology and biochemistry (see Table 4.3). Almost equally interesting is the question of why bacteria produce them in the first place. Sometimes this makes good sense, as when the cholera toxin induces copious watery diarrhoea, spreading the infection far and wide, but in other cases it seems fairly pointless, as when tetanus toxin kills the host by paralysing his nervous system. There are also bacterial enzymes that help their spread by breaking down tissues, streptococcal hyaluronidase being a typical example.

Exotoxins and endotoxins

There is an important distinction to be made between toxins actively secreted by the infectious organism, which are known as *exotoxins* (exo = outside) and others, known as *endotoxins* (endo = inside), that are part of its structure and are not released unless it dies. We will meet endotoxins again when considering immunopathology, because they have profound effects on the immune system (see Chapter 6), but they are not as dramatically toxic as most exotoxins. For example, it takes at least 100 μg of *Salmonella typhi* endotoxin to kill a mouse, whereas the same amount of *Clostridium botulinum* exotoxin will kill a million mice.

Table 4.3 Bacterial exotoxins and their mode of action

Example	Mode of action	Clinical result
Cholera E. coli [1] Salmonella[1]	Activates adenylate cyclase (without killing cells)	Loss of fluid and electrolytes from intestine; diarrhoea
C. perfringens	Lysis of cells by enzyme action (phospholipase)	Necrosis and spread ('gas gangrene')
Staph. aureus[2]	Lysis of cells by insertion of pores into membrane	Necrosis and spread; killing of phagocytes
Strep. pyogenes[2]	Lysis of connective tissue	Necrosis and spread
Diphtheria	Inhibition of protein synthesis	Respiratory tract damage; also heart, CNS
Tetanus (C. tetani)	Blocks inhibition of nerve–muscle transmission	Spastic paralysis
C. botulinum	Blocks acetylcholine release at nerve–muscle junction	Flaccid paralysis

[1] *These and other Gram-negative bacilli also contain endotoxins.*
[2] *Staphylococci and streptococci produce numerous exotoxins.*

Diarrhoea and vomiting

As everyone knows, the usual cause of acute diarrhoea and/or vomiting is eating or drinking something 'infected'. However, there is an important difference between very acute symptoms coming on within hours of eating (usually referred to as 'food poisoning') and those occurring a day or more later. In the former, it is likely that the food contained already formed exotoxins, which could therefore act at once. In the latter case, there were probably microorganisms present, but they had to multiply and colonize the intestine before producing symptoms ('gastroenteritis').

Table 4.4 shows examples of the two situations. Note that the treatment in each case would be somewhat different; while *fluid and electrolyte replacement* is the key in both, an infection with living organisms may call for antibiotics, whereas not much can be done about toxins (unless antitoxin is available, as it may be for botulism), and the combination of vomiting and diarrhoea usually serves to get rid of the toxin.

ENTRY AND ITS PREVENTION

A successful parasite must gain access to the site in which it intends to live. This may involve anything from merely clinging on firmly enough to some body surface to avoid being brushed or flushed away (as staphylococci and lice do on the skin, and many other organisms in the nose, throat, and intestine) to penetrating the body's most intimate areas (liver, blood, brain). In addition, if the parasite needs to spread to another host, it must have a

Table 4.4 Food poisoning and gastroenteritis compared

	Organism	Main source	Clinical effect
Food poisoning	*Staph. aureus*	Tinned and/or reheated food	Vomiting
	B. cereus		Vomiting, diarrhoea
	C. perfringens		Diarrhoea
	C. botulinum		Paralysis
Gastroenteritis	Viral		
	Rotavirus	Faecal–oral	Vomiting, diarrhoea
	Other viruses		
	Bacterial		
	Salmonella	Food	Diarrhoea
	Shigella		
	E. coli		
	Vibrio cholerae	Water	Watery diarrhoea
	Campylobacter		
	Yersinia		
	Protozoal		
	E. histolytica (amoebic dysentery)		Bloody diarrhoea
	Giardia		Chronic diarrhoea
	Cryptosporidium		

means of exit. Table 4.5 lists the main methods that parasites adopt for getting in and out of the body.

Larger animals have evolved many mechanisms to prevent this. The fact that wounds and burns readily get infected, mainly with bacteria, is a sign that the normal intact skin is an efficient barrier. In the same way, the repeated lung infections in patients with cystic fibrosis (see Chapter 1) indicate that the normal flushing of the bronchial tree by mucus and upwardly beating cilia is highly effective in keeping microorganisms out of the lower parts of the lung. Figure 4.1 shows these and other important external defences.

Table 4.5 The principal routes of entry and exit by infectious organisms

Entry	Examples	Exit
Skin contact	Smallpox, wart viruses, fungi, ectoparasites	Skin contact
Insect bite	Yellow fever, malaria[1]	Insect bite[2]
Animal bite	Rabies	–
Wound, burn	Staphylococci Tetanus, gas gangrene	– –

Inhalation	Respiratory viruses
	   Adeno-, rhino-, influenza,
	   measles, mumps, VZV
	 Bacteria
	   Tuberculosis, diphtheria,
	   anthrax, legionella
	 Fungi
	   Aspergillus, Histoplasma
		Coughing, sneezing

Food, water	Enteroviruses
	   Polio, Echo, hepatitis A
	 Bacteria
	   Salmonella, Shigella, cholera
	 Protozoa
	   Amoeba, Giardia
		Faeces (diarrhoea)[3]

Milk	*Brucella, Listeria*, tuberculosis	
Meat, fish	Tapeworms	–
Sexual contact	HIV, herpes 2, gonococcus, spirochaete	Sexual contact
Mother–fetus	Rubella, syphilis, HIV, malaria	
Needles, blood transfusion	Hepatitis B, HIV, malaria	

[1] *See Table 3.9 for a complete list.*
[2] *Not followed by further spread.*
[3] *See Table 4.4.*

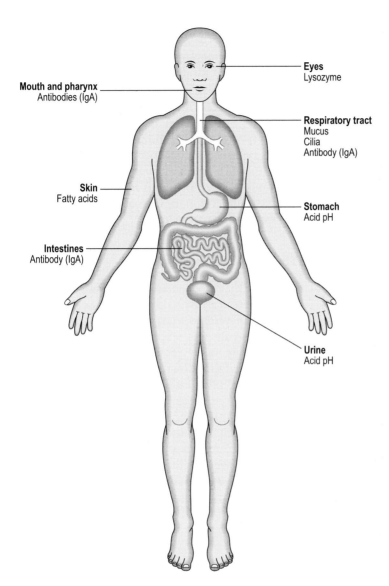

Eyes
Lysozyme

Mouth and pharynx
Antibodies (IgA)

Respiratory tract
Mucus
Cilia
Antibody (IgA)

Skin
Fatty acids

Stomach
Acid pH

Intestines
Antibody (IgA)

Urine
Acid pH

Fig. 4.1 The external defences of the body. The air we breathe, our skin and our intestinal tract are crowded with microbes. Most of these are bacteria and viruses, with occasional fungi, but in tropical countries protozoa and helminths (worms) add further to the burden. Bactericidal skin secretions, gastric acidity, and mucus and cilia in the bronchial tree help to reduce the load while intact epithelium generally keeps them from entering the tissues. In the blood and secretions, the enzyme lysozyme kills many bacteria by attacking their cell walls. IgA antibody is also important in the defence of mucous surfaces.

THE INFECTIOUS PERIOD; CARRIERS

In the normal course of most infections, the patient recovers, the responsible organisms having been eliminated by the immune system (see Chapter 6). Thus the period during which they can spread to another victim is fairly restricted, and an estimate of this is the basis for the *quarantine* period. Exactly how long this is will depend on many factors, including most of those in Table 4.1. But in certain cases the patient can recover without eliminating the infectious organisms; such people are called *carriers*, and create a problem, since through no fault of their own they can infect large numbers of others. Typhoid, gonorrhoea, and hepatitis B are three infections where healthy carriers are common. One obvious conclusion is that these are not caused by cytopathic organisms!

LOCAL AND SYSTEMIC INFECTION

Infectious organisms may or may not remain at their site of entry into the body. If they do, we suffer a *localized* infection at that site; examples would be a cold or sore throat from viruses that have attached to the mucous membrane of the nose or throat, or a staphylococcal infection of a skin wound. Often, however, the organism travels to some other site to set up residence: the hepatitis viruses to the liver, polio and rabies viruses to the central nervous system, etc. The infection is still localized, but to an internal organ. Sometimes an infection spreads in what appears to be an uncontrolled manner, as when staphylococci or tubercle bacilli get into the bloodstream and disseminate all over the body to become *systemic*, or a virulent streptococcus races through the tissues (the 'flesh-eating virus' so beloved of journalists). The presence in the blood of bacteria (bacteraemia) is usually an extremely dangerous sign, but virus particles are more common because many viruses spreading from their site of entry to an internal organ spend a brief period in the blood (viraemia).

WORM INFECTIONS

Because of their relatively enormous size, worms can cause special problems. A cricket-ball sized hydatid cyst or amoebic abscess in the liver, lung, or brain will produce the same symptoms as a large tumour – indeed, they are occasionally misdiagnosed as such. A filarial worm completely obstructing a lymphatic in the leg can lead to the massive oedema of elephantiasis (though this has an immunological component too). Other roundworms can obstruct the bile duct or the intestine, or migrate through the lungs triggering violent asthma. Hookworms in the intestine can deplete the patient of enough blood to cause severe anaemia. And so on.

FEVER

In many people's minds, a temperature is virtually synonymous with an infection. About 30–50% of cases of 'PUO' (pyrexia of unknown origin – that is, unexplained fever lasting 3 weeks or more) are due to infection, other major causes being chronic inflammatory disease (rheumatic, etc.) and cancer. However, most infections do cause fever, and occasionally the pattern is helpful in diagnosis; for example, the 2- or 3-day cycle of malaria, the swinging temperature of an abscess, the chronic low-grade fever of tuberculosis, or the relapsing pattern of brucellosis.

While it is true that a temperature of more than about 104°F (40°C) may sometimes need to be brought down for the patient's comfort (e.g. by cold sponging or antipyrexial drugs), fever is not in itself a danger to life unless it reaches about 107°F (41.5°C) or is due to external heating ('heat stroke'). It is in fact a resetting of the temperature regulating centre in the hypothalamus, triggered by normal communication molecules known as *cytokines* (see Chapter 5 for their role in immunity) with several possible benefits to the patient. Many defence mechanisms work faster at higher temperature, while some microorganisms may even be damaged – which was the rationale, earlier in this century, for treating syphilis with deliberate malaria infection.

FEELING ILL

Apart from fever, other general symptoms often tell you that you are ill. Tiredness, muscle pains, headache are a common feature of many infections. It is becoming clear that, like fever, they are due to higher than usual levels of the body's natural communication molecules such as interferons, interleukins, etc. (see *cytokines*, Chapter 5). In fact patients treated for cancer and other conditions with some of these substances are often convinced they are 'going down with flu'. It is perhaps some consolation to know that these unpleasant symptoms are due to the body's own defences going into action!

A FINAL WORD ON PATHOGENESIS

In this chapter we have mentioned many ways in which an infectious organism can produce disease, and there are more to come in Chapter 7 when we discuss immunopathology. However, it must be emphasized that in many infections we still do not really understand exactly why the patient becomes ill, and considerable research is nowadays focused on this question.

Tutorial 4

Try your hand at the following typical essay questions related to pathogenesis (the way organisms cause disease).

QUESTIONS

1. Some viruses kill their host cell, some do not. Discuss the significance of this.

2. Distinguish between exotoxins and endotoxins.

3. What might determine the period during which a patient is 'infectious'?

4. What is the use of fever?

5. How would it change your life if you were a carrier of (a) hepatitis B, (b) typhoid, or (c) nasal staphylococci?

ANSWERS

1. Viruses that kill their host cell are certain to damage tissue to some extent. Typical examples are influenza, cold viruses, polio. If they do not, they may be persistent, leading to the carrier state (e.g. hepatitis B) or they may become latent, causing no trouble until they are reactivated (e.g. chickenpox/shingles). If a non-destructive virus is to spread elsewhere in the body, it usually needs to be enveloped in host membrane. Because their envelopes contain molecules that bind to normal cells, they can spread from cell to cell without exposure to the 'outside', which has a significant effect on how the immune system responds. In contrast, enveloped viruses are less effective at person to person spread, especially by the intestinal route.

2. Exotoxins are secreted, highly toxic, usually protein. Endotoxins are cell wall components, mainly of Gram-negative bacteria, less toxic, acting mainly on the immune system, mainly non-protein (many are lipopolysaccharides). It is believed that bacterial exotoxins may have been one of the driving forces for the gradual evolution of the antibody response in vertebrates (see Chapter 5).

3. A patient is infectious as long as the offending organism can leave his body and infect another. This depends on whether, and how rapidly, the host defences can kill it (see Chapter 6 for a discussion of why immunity is effective in some infections and not in others). It also depends on how effective the organism is at setting up an infection in a new host. The organism must also have access to the outside, so it is favoured by coughing, sneezing, diarrhoea, close contact. In some protozoal and worm diseases spread by insects, only one particular stage of the parasite can be transmitted; this explains why malaria is mainly transmitted at night. You can see that 'infectious' is a relative term, and quarantine periods are based on experience rather than on strictly scientific principles.

4. Since the question does not specify which, you should consider 'usefulness' from all possible viewpoints. A raised temperature is thought to benefit many of the cellular and molecular processes involved in immunity (see Chapter 5). It also inclines the patient to lie down and rest the infected part, which probably reduces the chance of the disease spreading to others. Some infections may be inhibited at high temperature – though this has never really been proved, and some could actually grow more rapidly. So to the patient, fever is probably, in moderation, useful. To the doctor it is a sign that something is wrong, and if it lasts more than a week or so, it certainly needs investigating.

5. A carrier of hepatitis B should not be a blood donor, and should not work in 'exposure-prone' conditions where blood may be transmitted to others (e.g. dentistry, midwifery). Prolonged treatment with interferon (see Chapter 5) may be able to terminate the carrier state. A typhoid carrier should not work with food; the famous cook 'Typhoid Mary' is thought to have infected at least 200 people. As to nasal staphylococci, we are all carriers, but if you carry an antibiotic-resistant strain (see MRSA, Chapter 8) you should not come into contact with patients, particularly not surgical or immunodeficient ones, until you have been treated and pronounced clear.

FURTHER READING

There are a number of good comprehensive textbooks on infectious disease, most of them colourfully illustrated. Here is a selection:

Bannister B A, Begg N T 1996 Infectious disease. Blackwell Science, Oxford, 484 pp
Predominantly system-based.

Beeching N J, Cheesbrough J S 1994 Infectious diseases. Mosby Year Book, Mosby, London 126 pp
One of the Wolfe series, quiz-based, with illustrated case histories.

Ellner P D, Neu H C 1992 Understanding infectious disease. Mosby Year Book, Mosby, London 343 pp
American, system-based with short case histories.

Mandell G L, Bennett J E, Dolin R 1995 Principles and practice of infectious diseases, 4th edn. Churchill Livingstone, Edinburgh 2804 pp
American, multi-author.

Schaechter M, Medoff G, Eisenstein B I (eds) 1992 Mechanisms of microbial disease. Williams & Wilkins, Baltimore, 973 pp
A multi-author compendium of infectious organisms (viruses to worms) and how they cause disease.

Taussig M J 1984 Processes in pathology and microbiology, 2nd edn. Blackwell Scientific, Boston

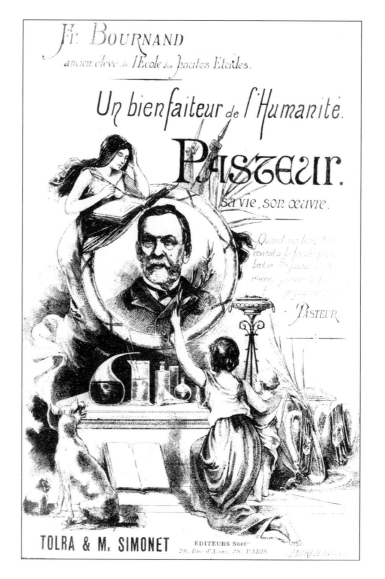

This frontispiece from a life of Louis Pasteur published in the year of his death (1895) illustrates the extraordinary level of adulation this great scientist inspired. Apart from his enormous contributions to the understanding of infection and immunity (it was Pasteur who proved that infection was always due to living organisms and could not be generated spontaneously), he made major advances in the chemical, beer, silk, and dairy industries; the heating of milk to sterilize it is still known as 'pasteurization'.

The immune system

5

■ CONTENTS

Case 5.1

In July 1885, the great French scientist Louis Pasteur performed his most daring experiment. A 9-year-old boy, Joseph Meister, had been bitten 14 times by a rabid dog 3 days earlier and was certain to die. Pasteur's work with dogs had shown that the spinal cord of rabid animals, dried for 2 weeks to 'inactivate' it, and injected as a suspension, could protect against otherwise fatal rabies following a subsequent injection of undried cord. Joseph was given 13 injections, and survived to become the first caretaker of the famous Pasteur Institute in Paris.

Considering that Pasteur did not know the cause of rabies (viruses were only discovered in 1900), that his treatment was applied *after* exposure, and that failure would have delighted his numerous enemies, his experiment was certainly courageous. The only real precedent he had to go on was the cowpox vaccine introduced by Jenner a century earlier and known to somehow induce immunity against smallpox. But other scientists were making discoveries that seemed to explain Pasteur's results. For instance, when inactivated diphtheria toxin was used as a vaccine against diphtheria, the protective effect was found to reside in a serum factor, which was baptized *antibody*. And when a transparent starfish was put under the microscope and injected with small splinters of wood, cells could be seen swarming to destroy and digest them, by a process that was termed *phagocytosis*. Thus by about 1900 it was understood that there was a set of cells and molecules in the body, specialized for dealing with foreign material, and that some of them, at least, could *learn* to respond more vigorously as a result of repeated exposure. All such cells and molecules came to be known as the *immune system*, and the science of immunology had begun.

Jumping ahead another hundred years, we can sum up the properties of the immune system as follows:

1. Some of its activities depend on molecules (e.g. antibody, complement, cytokines) that circulate in the blood and other body fluids. Others require the presence of intact cells (e.g. phagocytes, lymphocytes). In immunological jargon, immunity can be *humoral* or *cellular*.
2. Some of its components function in the same way throughout life (e.g. complement, phagocytes) while others display *memory*, or the ability to progressively adapt and learn from experience (e.g. antibody, lymphocytes). In immunological jargon, immunity can be *natural* or *adaptive*.
3. Some components are specialized mainly for *recognition* of foreign material, others for its *disposal*, and others again for *communication* between the various different cells involved.

With this introduction, let us look in more detail at the basic structure and function of the immune system, leaving its precise role in infectious disease for the following chapter, but always bearing in mind that the whole reason for its existence is to deal with infectious organisms.

NATURAL AND ADAPTIVE IMMUNITY

This is one of the most important distinctions to understand, because it explains many features of infections, such as: Why are some infections eliminated rapidly while others take weeks? Why do you only get some infections once but others repeatedly? How do vaccines work? What infections will occur in an immunodeficient patient? It also helps to explain several unfortunate phenomena such as allergy and the rejection of grafts.

Table 5.1 lists the essential features of natural and adaptive immunity. You will note that the cells and molecules of the natural immune system are the same as those involved in acute and chronic inflammation: neutrophils, macrophages, and complement (look back at Chapter 2), together with the cytokines already mentioned in Chapter 4. So as well as responding to damaged tissue and speeding up repair, they each have a role in eliminating infectious organisms, which of course often get in as a result of damage. Thus natural immunity acts as a first line of defence, rapid in its action, not very discriminating in what it attacks, but highly effective in keeping us free of infection most of the time.

In contrast, adaptive immunity depends on the activity of the lymphocyte – a relatively new type of cell in evolutionary terms, since it appeared only with the earliest vertebrates, about 500 million years ago (for the 1.5 billion years before that, animals managed with just natural immunity). Lymphocytes act slowly but with great precision, recognizing and remembering individual foreign organisms and even individual molecules derived from them, so that when they meet them again months or years later, they attack them more vigorously. This is what is referred to as *immunological memory*, and is seen very clearly in diseases like measles and mumps, where the first

Table 5.1 The natural and adaptive immune systems contrasted

	Natural	Adaptive
Cells	Phagocytes[1] 　Neutrophil 　Macrophage 　Eosinophil 　Mast cell; basophil 　Natural killer cell[1]	Lymphocytes[2] 　B lymphocyte 　T lymphocyte 　Helper 　Cytotoxic
Molecules ('humoral factors')	Complement[1] Cytokines (especially interferons) Acute phase proteins	Antibody[2] Cytokines (especially interleukins)
Speed and duration	Rapid, short-lived	Slow, prolonged, can increase
Development of memory	No	Yes
Present in	All animals	Vertebrates only

[1] These components have the ability to recognize foreign material with low specificity.
[2] These components have the ability to recognize foreign material with high specificity.

infection lasts a week or two but the second is 'nipped in the bud' so quickly that the patient never even becomes ill.

Natural and adaptive immunity seldom act in isolation. For example, it is very common for *B lymphocytes* to recognize, say, a bacterium, and make *antibody* which binds to the bacterium and helps a *phagocyte* to engulf it. When you think that the lymphocyte may have needed help from a *T lymphocyte* to make the antibody, while the phagocytosis can be further speeded up by *complement*, you will appreciate that the immune system is really an integrated whole, rather like the brain, with different elements becoming more important in different situations.

CELLS OF THE IMMUNE SYSTEM

The cells of the immune system form part of the haemopoietic system – that is, they originate from precursors in the bone marrow and spend a variable part of their lives in the bloodstream and the various lymphoid organs and tissues. In contrast to the red cells (erythrocytes), the white blood cells are called leucocytes and have quite different shapes and sizes when viewed under the microscope (Fig. 5.1).

The natural immune system

Phagocytic cells

We have already mentioned the polymorphs in Chapter 2. These mobile phagocytic cells, so called because of their multilobed nuclear shape, stain

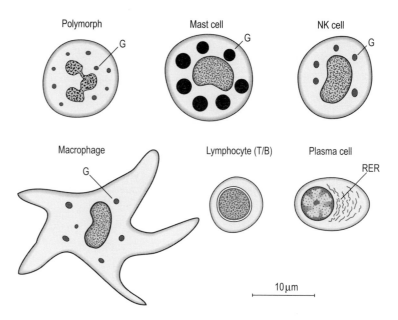

Fig. 5.1 Cells of the immune response. Polymorphs are the most common white blood cells. Macrophages derived from blood-borne monocytes are found in all the tissues of the body. Both polymorphs and macrophages are phagocytic and have small granules (G) in their cytoplasm containing cytotoxic substances. Mast cells with their large granules containing pharmacologically active chemicals are present in the connective tissues, especially those beneath epithelial surfaces. Here they play a role in the acute inflammatory response. Natural killer (NK) cells are found mostly in the bloodstream but also in the tissues, and are our first cellular line of defence against viruses. They also have large granules containg cytotoxic molecules. The majority of lymphocytes (B and T) are found in lymphoid tissues/organs. Plasma cells are B cells with the cellular structures (rough endoplasmic reticulum: RER) required for synthesis of large amounts of antibody.

with neutral dyes and are therefore called neutrophils. Other granulocytes stain with basic dyes (basophils) or with eosin (eosinophils). Neutrophils are the most abundant granulocytes in the circulation (around 90%). They are produced in large numbers in the bone marrow (10^8/day) and they have a short life of only a few days – dying by the process of apoptosis (see Chapter 2). As already mentioned, these cells are major players in the acute inflammatory response and emigrate from the bloodstream in response to chemotactic stimuli. As we will see later (Chapter 6), different immune cells function against different infectious organisms. Neutrophils are particularly efficient at dealing with bacteria that live in the tissues but not inside cells.

Macrophages are also phagocytic and are derived from circulating blood monocytes. Unlike the neutrophils that migrate out of the bloodstream to carry out their function, they are resident in all tissues of the body (even the brain!) and form part of the 'mononuclear phagocyte' system. Together with the lymphocytes, monocytes are termed 'mononuclear' to distinguish them by shape from the neutrophils with their multilobed nucleus. Examples of these mononuclear phagocytes in different sites of the body are shown in Figure 5.2. Carbon particles (or bacteria) injected intravenously

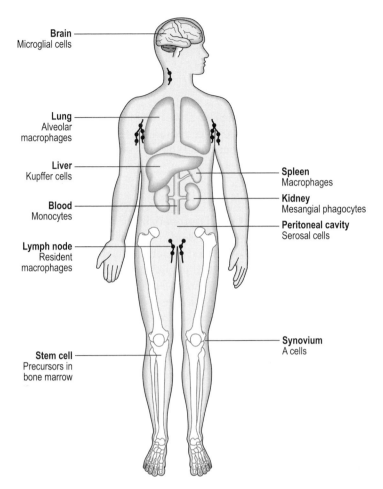

Brain
Microglial cells

Lung
Alveolar
macrophages

Liver
Kupffer cells

Blood
Monocytes

Lymph node
Resident
macrophages

Stem cell
Precursors in
bone marrow

Spleen
Macrophages

Kidney
Mesangial phagocytes

Peritoneal cavity
Serosal cells

Synovium
A cells

Fig. 5.2 Cells of the mononuclear phagocyte system. Macrophages are found in the alveoli (alveolar macrophages) and in the brain (microglial cells). Kupffer cells line the sinusoidal spaces of the liver and mesangial cells are present in the glomeruli of the kidney. Serosal cells line the wall of the peritoneal cavity. The spleen and the many lymph nodes contain macrophages. 'A' cells in the synovial membranes of synovial joints are also members of this system. All these cells are derived from the pool of circulating monocytes produced from stem cell precursors in the bone marrow.

into mice localize in those tissues and organs containing the most phagocytic cells, demonstrating the extent of this phagocytic 'network'. It seems likely that macrophages are absolutely essential for existence, since there have been no reports of 'immunodeficiency' diseases where these cells fail to develop, unlike those described for neutrophils and lymphocytes (Chapter 7). Macrophages, like neutrophils, kill phagocytosed microbes by oxygen-dependent (involving hydrogen peroxide and oxygen free radicals) and oxygen-independent mechanisms (involving lysozyme and cationic proteins). As well as playing a role in phagocytosis, macrophages are important in chronic inflammation and subsequently in tissue reorganization by secretion of a number of enzymes, e.g. collagenase, and growth factors including fibroblast-stimulating factors and angiogenesis factors for stimulating the development of new blood vessels (see Chapter 2). Macrophages also work together with T lymphocytes in the adaptive immune response (see below).

Eosinophils, comprising 2–5% of the blood leucocytes, also have a phagocytic function but mainly seem to be important in dealing with non-phagocytosable large parasites such as worms by release of toxins (e.g. major basic protein). They are also frequently found at inflammatory sites where they are believed to counteract the effects of histamine released from mast cells and basophils (see later).

Mast cells and basophils

Basophils are found in very small numbers in the circulation (< 0.2%). They are very similar to their tissue-localized counterparts, the mast cells, which are found in subcutaneous sites and generally in the connective tissues of the body, especially those beneath the epithelial layers in close proximity to the outside world, e.g. in the intestinal and respiratory tracts. These cells are characterized by large dense granules (see Fig. 5.1) containing pharmacologically active substances such as heparin (an anticoagulant) and histamine, which when released give rise to an acute inflammatory response. 'Degranulation' of large numbers of these cells can result in life-threatening situations in patients with allergies (see Chapter 7).

Natural killer (NK) cells

Natural killer cells are found in the circulation (5–15% of the lymphocyte-like cells) and in most tissues, where their primary function is to deal with virus-infected cells and possibly tumours (see Chapter 6). They are slightly larger than the true lymphocytes and have small granules in their cytoplasm containing substances responsible for the death of the infected cells they attack. Hence they are often referred to as large granular lymphocytes.

The adaptive immune system

Lymphocytes, so called because they were first identified in lymph, are quite different from the cells of the natural immune system in that they confer specificity and memory on the immune system. They are present in the bloodstream (around 1–2 million per ml) and in the organs and tissues of the lymphoid system. In general, lymphocytes are small rounded cells with little cytoplasm. The two main subpopulations of lymphocytes, the T and B lymphocytes, are morphologically identical but functionally very different. Unlike the cells of the natural immune system they carry specific surface molecules (usually referred to as receptors) which enable them to recognize individual foreign antigens. 'Antigen' is the general term given to any molecule to which an immune response can be made.

T lymphocytes

The T lymphocytes (also called T cells) are produced in the *thymus*, which is called a *primary* lymphoid organ. There are two kinds of these cells, which have different functions. Helper T cells (Th) have a surface molecule called CD4 or T4. The Th are pivotal cells which help most of the other cells of the immune system. They do this mainly by secreting 'cytokines' or 'interleukins' – the hormones of the immune system (see below). Since the AIDS virus (HIV) attacks these cells it is not surprising that the immune system becomes compromised, leaving the body open to infection (see Chapter 7). Cytotoxic T cells (Tc) can really be regarded as 'specific' NK cells. They have CD8 or T8 surface molecules instead of CD4 and have a similar function to NK cells, in that they kill cells infected with intracellular microbes such as viruses.

B lymphocytes

The primary lymphoid source of the B lymphocytes is the *bone-marrow*. The function of B lymphocytes is to produce antibodies which specifically attach to antigens on invading microbes. When they secrete a large amount of antibody they are called plasma cells (Fig. 5.1). They also have antibody molecules on their surface which function as their antigen receptors. This 'marker' allows us to distinguish them from T cells, which have their own specific antigen receptors and either CD4 or CD8 (see above). CD4, CD8, and antibody are just three of the hundreds of surface molecules that can be identified on the surface of cells by fluorescent dyes coupled to specific *monoclonal antibodies* (see below).

MOLECULES OF THE IMMUNE SYSTEM

Complement

This is a cascade system of molecules, similar in nature to the clotting, fibrinolytic and kinin systems which are all involved in the process of acute inflammation and tissue repair (see Fig. 2.1). Complement is composed of around 20 proteins, some of which are present in relatively large quantities in the circulation (e.g. C3: 1.3 mg/ml). This latter component is the most important molecule in the complement system. To function, C3 has to be 'cleaved'. This can be brought about in two ways. The first occurs spontaneously on the surface of certain bacteria and is helped by other molecules such as properdin. This is termed the 'alternative pathway', since it was discovered more recently than the 'classical pathway', which involves molecules of the adaptive immune system – antibodies. In the classical pathway the C3 molecule is cleaved following the binding of antibody to an antigen. Activation of C3 by either pathway leads to further components having biological activity. The three main functions of complement and the components initiating them are illustrated in Table 5.2.

Cytokines

The cells of the immune system described above do not work independently but usually act together to produce their effects. This interaction is orchestrated by small proteins called cytokines produced by a variety of cells but mostly by lymphocytes and macrophages which act as communication

Table 5.2 Components of complement and their main functions

Complement components	Biological effects
C3a, C5a	Attracts neutrophils and causes mast cells to degranulate Results in *inflammation*
C3b	Attaches microbe to phagocyte (opsonization) leading to greatly enhanced *phagocytosis*
C5–C9	Attack the membrane of the microbe by punching a hole in it Results in death by *lysis* of the microbe

molecules between cells of the immune system. They function mainly over short distances but some can work over large distances, behaving like the 'hormones' of the immune system. Table 5.3 lists the main cytokines and what they do. As you will see, they have a wide range of functions with some confusing nomenclature.

Some are called *interleukins* (prefixed by IL, Latin for 'between leucocytes') but others, although having similar functions, do not conform to this

Table 5.3 Principal sources of cytokines and their main functions

Cells	Cytokines	Main function
Macrophages	IL1, TNF-α	T, B cell activation, fever Inflammation, fever
Monocytes	GCSF MCSF	Granulocyte growth Monocyte growth
T lymphocytes	IL2 IL3 IL4 IL5 IL6 IL7 IL8 IL9 IL10 IL13 TGF-β TNF-β IFN-γ	T, B cell growth Growth of cells (many types) B cell growth B, eosinophil growth B cell stimulation, production of APP Early B cell development Attraction of monos, PMN Growth of mast cells Inhibits other cytokines Like IL4, inhibits IFN-γ Inhibits other cytokines Inflammation, fever Antiviral, activates macrophages
Many cells	IL12 GMCSF IFN-α IFN-β	Stimulates T and NK cells Granulocyte and monocyte growth Antiviral Antiviral

IL: interleukin; TNF: tumour necrosis factor; GMCSF: granulocyte/monocyte colony stimulating factor; TGF: transforming growth factor; IFN: interferon.

nomenclature. They function to attract neutrophils and monocytes (e.g. IL8); enhance the development of T cell and B cell function (e.g. IL2, IL4); promote growth of cells in the bone marrow (e.g. granulocyte monocyte colony stimulating factor – GMCSF), which can result in a massive increase in blood neutrophils in acute bacterial infections; induce the production of acute phase proteins mainly by liver cells (e.g. IL6). Some cytokines, when produced in excess, may also contribute to tissue damage (e.g. tumour necrosis factor – TNF), and this will be discussed in Chapter 7.

Interferons (IFN) are also thought of as cytokines and are produced by all cells that have been infected with viruses. Most nucleated cells of the body produce IFN-α and IFN-β. Production of interferon prevents the spread of viral infections to neighbouring cells. T lymphocytes and NK cells produce a different type of interferon (IFN-γ) as part of their function in the adaptive and natural immune responses respectively (see immune responses, below).

Acute phase proteins (APP) are part of the body's immediate response to almost any injury or infection. Made in the liver, some of them rise dramatically in concentration (e.g. C-reactive protein – a 1000-fold increase), whilst others increase only modestly (e.g. fibrinogen by a factor of 2–4). There is an increase in the same order of the complement components C3 and C4, which can therefore also be considered as APP.

Antibodies

These are specific glycoproteins made by B cells and plasma cells whose function is to attach to microbial antigens and 'mark' them for disposal by the phagocytic cells, NK cells, and complement of the natural immune system. They occur in milligram quantities in the blood and tissues. They are composed of four polypeptide chains arranged into domain structures as shown in Figure 5.3. The antibody molecule has an antigen binding region (actually 2 antigen binding sites) called the $F(ab)_2$, whilst the other end of the molecule, the Fc, is involved in the biological functions (e.g. complement activation, attachment to phagocytes). There are five main *classes* of antibodies, each having particular biological activities (Table 5.4). Although they are all generally found in the bloodstream they predominate at different sites of the body depending on their major function. Because they are globular proteins, antibodies are often referred to as immuno-globulins (Ig). Antibodies and complement mainly deal with extracellular microbes and both can contribute to efficient phagocytosis (opsonization, see Chapter 2).

Major histocompatibility molecules

As we will be discussing in more detail later, the function of the immune system is to recognize foreign microbes and then dispose of them. Recognition by B cells is fairly straightforward: their surface antibody molecules recognize the shape of individual antigens. T lymphocytes, how-ever, cannot recognize large protein antigens unless they have been broken down ('processed') into smaller pieces of peptides by cellular enzymes. The molecules which attach to and 'present' these peptides to the T cells are

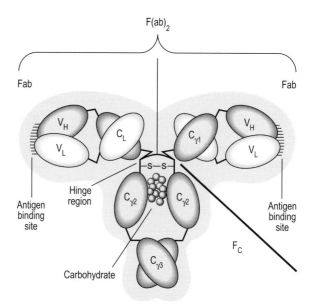

Fig. 5.3 Structure of antibodies. A typical antibody molecule is composed of two units of polypeptide chains (one heavy and one light) held together by covalent disulphide bonds. These peptides form 'domain' structures by the formation of uniform intrachain disulphide bonds. As determined from crystallographic studies, two of these identical heavy and light chains are held together by disulphide bonds to form the secondary structure shown. One end of the molecule contains two antigen binding sites (the F(ab)$_2$ region), whilst the biological activity of the molecule involved in complement fixation, opsonization, etc., is at the other end (Fc region). Variation in the amino acid sequence in the VH and VL domain determines the specificity of the molecule. There are two types of light chain – kappa and lambda – and five major types of heavy chain which determine the antibody class – IgM-μ, IgG-γ, IgA-α, IgD-δ and IgE-ε. These have different predominant biological activities (see Table 5.4). The antibody shown in this figure is IgG. (After J.H.L. Playfair and P.M. Lydyard, *Medical Immunology for Students*, Churchill Livingstone, Edinburgh, 1996.)

Table 5.4 The five classes of antibodies

Class	Size (kDa)	Main location	Biological activity
IgM	900	Blood	Agglutinates microbes; activates C'
IgG[1]	150	Blood and tissues	Acts as an opsonin; activates C'; important in ADCC; only Ig to cross the placenta
IgA	160	Mucosal surfaces	Agglutinates microbes; protected from proteolysis; secreted into lumen of gut, eye, etc.
IgE	180	Subepithelial tissues	Enhances acute inflammation by causing mast cell degranulation; important in allergy
IgD	180	On surface of B cells only	Thought to be involved in 'activation' of B cells

C': complement; Ig: immunoglobulin; ADCC; antibody-dependent cellular cytotoxicity.
[1] There are four subclasses of IgG (IgG1–4) with slightly different functions.

known as the major histocompatibility molecules (MHC). This may seem a strange name to call molecules with this function, but historically they were first identified by immunologists in the mid-1940s as being the antigens themselves which are responsible for the rejection of transplanted tissues and organs in mice such as skin, kidney, heart, and liver – hence histo(tissue) compatibility. In man they were first found on leucocytes and are therefore called human leucocyte antigens or HLA, and we shall use this term from now on. We now know that there are two main classes of HLA which have the function of displaying pieces of the microbe at the surface of an infected cell. HLA class I molecules HLA-A, B, or C are present on all nucleated cells of the body and present pieces of the virus infecting a cell. HLA class II molecules HLA-D (further subdivided into DR, DQ, or DP), on the other hand, are only found on certain cells, namely those with which Th cells may need to interact: e.g. B cells, macrophages and specialized *antigen-presenting* cells in the lymphoid tissues and skin (e.g. Langerhans cells)

ANATOMY OF THE IMMUNE SYSTEM

We have already mentioned that many of the cells involved in immunity are present in the bloodstream. These include the neutrophils, basophils and eosinophils, the monocytes (macrophage precursors), NK cells and lymphocytes. The phagocyte system has already been described (see Fig. 5.2). The lymphocytes also have their own 'system' – the lymphoid system. They are produced in the primary lymphoid organs – the thymus and bone marrow – but then carry out their function in the secondary lymphoid organs and tissues (Fig. 5.4). The secondary lymphoid tissues include the spleen, lymph nodes ('glands'), and the abundant lymphoid tissues associated with the gut and other mucous surfaces The spleen, as well as being a lymphoid organ, is also important for the storage of red blood cells and the removal of old ones. There are lymph nodes throughout the body. You will be aware of the ones in your neck when you have a throat infection, or in the armpit following an infected finger. Each kind of secondary lymphoid tissue has a particular protective function – the spleen protects us against blood-borne microbes by acting as a blood filter and the lymph nodes drain the tissue spaces and therefore protect us against microbes entering the body through the skin, etc. However, by far the majority of the lymphoid tissue is found in the lining layers of the digestive, respiratory, and genitourinary tracts, which are the major portals of entry of microbes into the body. Here, the lymphoid tissue is found beneath the epithelial cells, many of which secrete mucus into the lumen of the tracts. The basic structure of the different secondary lymphoid tissues is seen in Figure 5.5. The T and B lymphocytes do not reside permanently in the different lymphoid tissues but continuously circulate around the body. It is estimated that they 'recirculate' through the different sites, including the bloodstream, about three times every day! (Fig. 5.6). They do this in search of microbes which they recognize through their specific antigen receptors. You can imagine that, without this recirculation, a microbe and its specific lymphocyte might never meet.

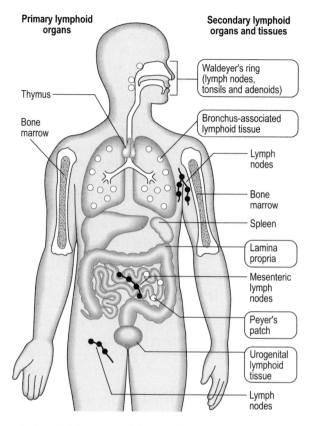

Primary lymphoid organs

Secondary lymphoid organs and tissues

- Thymus
- Bone marrow
- Waldeyer's ring (lymph nodes, tonsils and adenoids)
- Bronchus-associated lymphoid tissue
- Lymph nodes
- Bone marrow
- Spleen
- Lamina propria
- Mesenteric lymph nodes
- Peyer's patch
- Urogenital lymphoid tissue
- Lymph nodes

Fig. 5.4 The major lymphoid organs and tissues. The two primary lymphoid organs – sites of lymphocyte development – and the many secondary lymphoid organs/tissues – sites of lymphocyte function – are shown in this figure. The mucosa-associated secondary lymphoid tissue (MALT) is shown in boxes. This represents the majority of the overall lymphoid tissue and is located at the main entry points of microbes into the body. (After J.H.L. Playfair and P.M. Lydyard, *Medical Immunology for Students*, Churchill Livingstone, Edinburgh, 1996.)

RECOGNITION AND RECEPTORS

The immune system is designed to first recognize and then dispose of microbes. The recognition of microbes by the cells and molecules of the natural immune system is relatively *non-specific* – that is, one cell can recognize thousands of different microbes. This is in contrast to the more specific cell-surface and secreted antigen receptors of the adaptive immune system (Table 5.5). Although it is difficult to give an exact figure, it is estimated that there are at least 10–100 million different antibody specificities and about the same number of different T lymphocyte receptors. To give you some idea of the actual size of the antigen molecule recognized by the receptors, it is about six monosaccharides or 15 to 20 amino acids on a protein for antibodies, and 9 to 15 amino acids for the T cell receptor. Note that antigen receptors do not attach to microbial antigens by chemical bonding, but

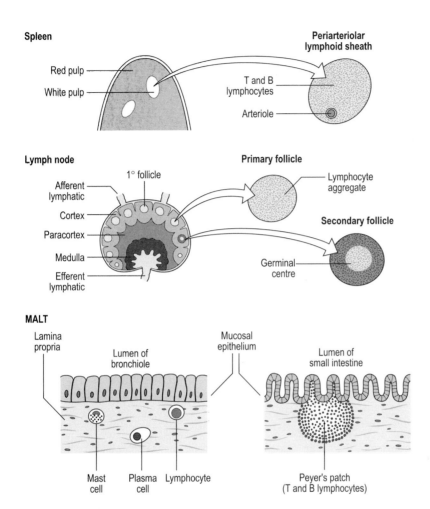

Fig. 5.5 Secondary lymphoid organs and tissues. Spleen: The white pulp contains T and B lymphocytes which respond to microbial antigens in the bloodstream. The lymphoid tissue surrounds an arteriole and is often called the periarteriolar lymphoid sheath (PALS). Lymph node: The many lymph nodes/glands drain the tissue spaces. Tissue fluid/lymph passes into the node via afferent lymphatic vessels into the cortex in which B cells are mostly arranged into aggregates (1° follicles). When these cells react to an antigen they proliferate to produce a 'germinal centre'. This is then termed a 2° follicle. The T lymphocytes are found mostly in the paracortex and T and B lymphocytes and plasma cells in the medulla. Mucosa-associated tissue (MALT): lymphocytes and plasma cells (and mast cells) are found in the connective tissue beneath the mucosal surfaces (lamina propria). Large aggregates of lymphocytes beneath the mucosal surface are also seen in the lower intestine (Peyer's patches).

rather through physical forces including hydrogen bonds, electrostatic and Van der Waals forces. The fact that the cells of the natural immune system carry receptors for antibodies and complement, while lymphocytes have receptors for many cytokines, helps to explain how it is that all these immune elements work so efficiently together.

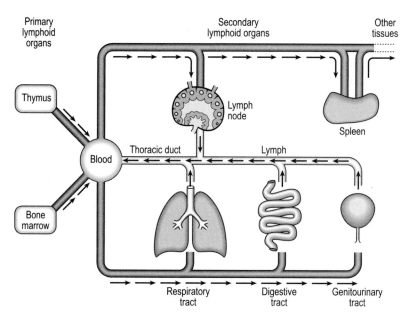

Fig. 5.6 Lymphocyte traffic. Lymphocytes produced in the primary lymphoid organs (thymus (T) and bone marrow (B)) migrate through the blood to the secondary lymphoid organs/tissues where they carry out their function. Many of the lymphocytes do not remain in these tissues but pass through the lymphatic system back into the circulation via a large collecting vessel, the thoracic duct. This empties into the venous bloodstream close to the heart.

Table 5.5 Cell-surface receptors of the immune system

Receptors	Structures recognized
Natural immune system	
Complement	Some bacteria (alternative pathway)
	Antibody bound to antigen (classical pathway)
Phagocytes	
Receptors for mannose	Some bacteria
Receptors for complement	Microbes covered with C3b
Receptors for antibodies	Microbes covered with IgG antibodies
C-reactive protein	Some bacteria
NK cell receptors	Cell surface structures altered by virus infection (not via HLA)
Mast cells	
Receptors for antibodies	Antigens covered with IgE antibodies
Adaptive immune system	
B lymphocytes	
Cell surface antibody	All microbial antigens
Antibodies released by plasma cells	All microbial antigens
T lymphocytes	
T cell receptor	Peptides presented by HLA
Antigen-presenting cells	
HLA molecules	T lymphocyte receptor

SPECIFICITY AND CLONAL SELECTION

The very large number of lymphocytes, each with its specific surface receptor, is necessary because there is such a wide variety of different microbes to be recognized. In fact each microbe carries many different antigens, in the form of surface proteins or sugars, and it is these antigens that 'select' which lymphocytes are brought into the immune response. Thus different microbes with different antigens will select different lymphocytes to mount a response. Attachment of the antigens to the receptors triggers a sequence of biochemical events which leads to cell division (proliferation), resulting in a large number of cells bearing the same specific receptor. This lymphocyte with its specific antigen receptor and its progeny is called a 'clone' and all cells within the clone have the same antigen specificity. Therefore lymphocytes taking part in an immune response are said to do so by 'clonal selection'. In Figure 5.7 we have shown two such clones, but in reality several hundred clones (both T and B) would be stimulated in a typical immune response. Two types of cells are produced following their stimulation, one which has an immediate effect on the microbe ('effector' cells) and the other termed 'memory' cells, which are kept in reserve for a future response to the same antigen. There are hundreds of cells in a particular clone, which comprise both effector and memory cells. The effector cells of B lymphocyte clones are the antibody-secreting plasma cells, whilst the

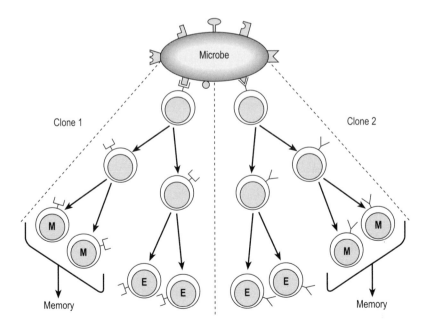

Fig. 5.7 Clonal selection of lymphocytes by antigens. Microbes have many different antigens. In this figure, two B lymphocytes are shown, each recognizing one antigen through its specific receptor and dividing to produce a clone of cells with identical receptors, some of which become memory cells (M) and some effector cells (E). The effector cells produced by B lymphocytes are the plasma cells, which secrete antibody into the blood. Note that in the case of T cells the microbial antigens have first to be 'processed' and presented by antigen-presenting cells, and that the effector cells would be either Th or Tc or both.

effector cells of T lymphocyte clones are cytotoxic or cytokine-secreting cells. It is through the memory cells that the immune system produces a much faster and more effective immune ('secondary') response to a microbe that it has previously encountered and eliminated. In the case of B cells the memory cells are produced in the germinal centres of the secondary follicles (see Fig. 5.5).

Tolerance or antigen unresponsiveness

Since some of the lymphocytes produced in the primary lymphoid organs/tissues will also have receptors for self antigens, these have to be eliminated or kept in check, otherwise they could produce disastrous effects. Fortunately the body has several different ways of preventing this (collectively termed 'self-tolerance'). The first is to eliminate the cells in the primary lymphoid organs when they are immature, and in fact many cells are known to die in these sites (thymus, bone marrow). Secondly, those cells that escape into the secondary lymphoid tissues, although able to recognize self antigens, can be prevented from actually producing effector and memory cells in a number of ways which are not fully understood. A few self antigens are restricted to sites which do not come into contact with the immune cells – e.g. eye proteins – and when they do, they produce an 'autoimmune response' (see Chapter 7).

IMMUNE RESPONSES

Even if the natural immune system is able to deal effectively with an invading microbe, the adaptive system is usually alerted. During an acute inflammatory response small numbers of lymphocytes will be exposed directly to the microbe (B lymphocytes) or pieces of microbe processed by antigen-presenting cells (T lymphocytes). This leads to stimulation of the two arms of the adaptive immune response: (a) antibody responses and (b) cell-mediated responses.

The antibody response

Specific antibodies can be detected in the bloodstream within a couple of days of first contact of a microbe with the immune system (the *primary* response). Their concentration increases over the next few days, reaches a peak and then decreases back to low levels (Fig. 5.8). By this time the antibodies – mainly IgM – should have carried out their function of eliminating the microbe through complement-mediated lysis, or opsonization and disposal by phagocytes. Exposure to the same microbe at a later date results in a *secondary* response, in which antibodies are produced more rapidly, there are more of them, and more of the other classes of antibody are produced, for example IgG. Furthermore, the antibodies have a higher 'affinity' for the antigens – that is, they 'fit' better and bind more strongly. Memory cells produced as the result of first contact with the microbe (Fig. 5.7) provide the cellular basis for the more rapid and larger secondary response. Memory cells are relatively long-lived, some surviving for several years,

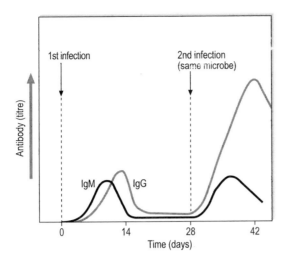

Fig. 5.8 The antibody response. Antibodies are detected in the blood soon after infection with a microbe. They increase, reach a peak, and then decrease. IgM antibodies are produced first, followed by IgG. If the same microbe infects again there is a more rapid, larger response, with IgG (and other classes) being more prominent. This will also reach a peak in the blood and then decrease. During the primary response, specific memory cells are produced which then lead to the qualitatively and quantitatively better secondary response (see text).

and further contact with the same microbe stimulates them once again to produce an effective response. It is this memory response which provides the theoretical basis for immunity to diseases such as measles and for vaccination (Chapter 6). As already noted, many different B lymphocyte clones are brought into the antibody response. It is technically possible to isolate individual clones of B cells making 'monoclonal' antibodies of a single specificity. Since monoclonal antibodies are highly specific they have a number of uses in medicine, including identification of microbes, identification of different cell types, 'imaging' of tumours, and even a therapeutic potential for specifically targeting toxins to microbes and tumours.

Cell-mediated response

'Cell-mediated immunity' is an old term used to denote all immune responses not directly involving antibodies. It is now generally applied to the two types of T-cell responses which are generated to deal specifically with intracellular microbes. (Remind yourself of which microbes are intracellular and which extracellular by reviewing Chapter 3.)

I. T cell 'help' for macrophages infected with microbes

Many microbial species entering a macrophage through the phagocytic pathway will be killed. In some cases, however, the microbes resist being killed and may persist within the phagocyte (see Chapter 6). Even so, small numbers of the microbe will die in the macrophage and be degraded by proteolytic enzymes. Pieces of the microbe (peptides) are then carried by

HLA Class II molecules to the cell membrane to show specific helper T cells (Th: CD4+) that they are infected and that they are required to get rid of the microbe (Fig. 5.9). T cells specific for the peptides will attach to them through their receptors and be stimulated to divide and produce the cytokine IFN-γ. The IFN-γ activates the killing mechanisms of the macrophage, resulting in elimination of the microbes.

Note that some helper T cells also help B lymphocytes to make antibodies. They do this by producing cytokines such as IL4 which act as a growth factor for B cells and others that help the B cells to develop into plasma cells (Fig. 5.1).

2. Cytotoxic T cells to kill virus-infected cells

Viruses can only survive and reproduce within nucleated cells. A virus infects a cell through binding to a specific surface receptor which acts as a door into the cell. Once inside, it starts to utilize the protein synthetic machinery of the cell to reproduce itself. Small pieces of the virus are accessible to proteolytic enzymes which degrade them into peptides (Fig. 5.9). These peptides are displayed on the surface of the infected cell to indicate to cytotoxic T cells (Tc: CD8+) that they are infected. Specific Tc bind through their receptors to the peptides (in this case presented with HLA Class I molecules) and go on to kill both cell and virus.

In the next chapter we look at how immunity to different types of infection is achieved using the processes outlined in this chapter.

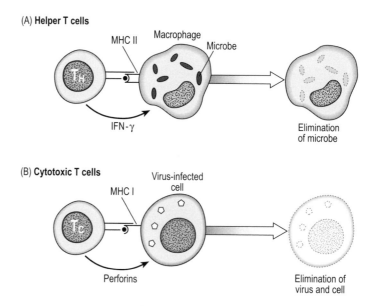

Fig. 5.9 Two types of cell-mediated responses. Helper T cells (Th) recognize peptides on the surface of macrophages infected with bacteria. They produce IFN-γ, which activates the killing mechanisms of the macrophage, thus eliminating the intracellular microbe. Cytotoxic T cells (Tc) recognize peptides derived from viruses infecting any nucleated body cell. They produce substances, e.g. perforins, which kill the infected cells.

FURTHER READING

There are many immunology textbooks of differing complexity.

Alberts B, Bray D, Lewis J, Raff M, Roberts K, Watson J D 1994 Molecular biology of the cell, 3rd edn. Garland, New York
Section on basic immunology.

Janeway C A Jr, Travers P 1996 Immunobiology, 2nd edn. Garland, New York
Easily digestible text with colourful explanatory diagrams.

Kuby J 1994 Immunology, 2nd edn. Freeman, Oxford
Good reference book with Scientific American style pictures.

Playfair J H L 1996 Immunology at a glance, 6th edn. Blackwell Science, Oxford
A simple introduction to the subject, half text and half figures.

Playfair J H L, Lydyard P M 1995 Medical immunology for students. Churchill Livingstone, Edinburgh
A core immunology text detailing basic immunology, immunopathology, and clinical immunology for medical students.

Roitt I M 1994 Essential immunology, 8th edn. Blackwell Scientific, Oxford
Top-selling immunology book in the UK, a good reference book for details.

Roitt I M, Brostoff J, Male D 1996 Immunology, 4th edn. Mosby, London
Well-illustrated basic immunology book.

Staines N, Brostoff J, James K 1993 Introducing immunology, 2nd edn. Mosby, London
A short, easy to understand pocket book illustrating basic principles.

Tutorial 5

QUESTIONS

1. What are the cells of the natural and adaptive immune systems? How do they differ from one another?

2. What are cytokines and what are their main functions?

3. What are monoclonal antibodies? How can they be used as diagnostic and therapeutic agents?

4. Why do lymphoid cells need to circulate around the body? How do they do it?

5. How do T cells know whether to 'kill' or 'help' cells infected with microbes?

6. How does the adaptive immune system 'remember' that it has previously encountered a specific microbe?

ANSWERS

1. The main cells of the natural immune system are the phagocytic cells – neutrophils (mobile in the bloodstream) and macrophages (in the tissues), the mast cells and the natural killer cells. The lymphocytes (T and B, produced in the thymus and bone marrow respectively) are the cells of the adaptive immune system. The main differences between the cells of the two systems are that the lymphocytes proliferate, recirculate, and display high antigen specificity and memory.

2. Cytokines are communication molecules. The main producer is the T cell but they can be produced by many different kinds of cells, in both the natural and adaptive systems. They can protect cells from viruses (e.g. interferons), attract neutrophils and monocytes (e.g. IL8; note that complement components can also do this), help T and B lymphocytes proliferate and develop into effector cells (e.g. IL2, IL4, IL6).

3. A monoclonal antibody (McAb) is the product of a single B cell clone. Each McAb is highly specific and therefore can be used to identify a specific antigen. Since different microbes have antigens peculiar to them, McAbs can be used to identify them (e.g. bacterial species and even their 'serotypes'). For this, McAb can be labelled with molecules which light up in the ultraviolet microscope (e.g. fluorescein). They can also be made against HLA molecules for tissue typing, used to identify different kinds of cells in pathological specimens, including tumours (immunohistochemistry), or labelled with radioisotopes to locate and characterize tumours in vivo (imaging) and even experimentally to kill the tumours, by virtue of the fact that radioactive substances are toxic to dividing cells (immunotherapy).

4. Each T and B cell has a specific receptor for a single antigen, with a total repertoire probably exceeding 10^8 different specificities. Each microbe has a limited number of antigens, and, in order to maximize the chance that a specific lymphocyte will come into contact with these antigens, many of the lymphocytes pass from the bloodstream into the different secondary lymphoid organs or tissues and back again, 'searching' for their specific antigens. Lymphocyte migration out of the bloodstream is mediated by specific 'adhesion molecules' which allow them to attach to and pass out between specialized capillary endothelial cells. Mucosal lymphocytes have special adhesion or 'homing' molecules which enable lymphocytes activated at one mucosal site to return to other mucosal tissues and carry out their function there.

5. T lymphocytes protect us against intracellular microbes. They recognize that a cell is infected by microbial antigens displayed on the surface (like a 'shop window'). Viruses 'hijack' the protein synthesis machinery of the cell and new viral proteins are digested into peptides which attach to the HLA Class I molecules and are placed at the surface membrane. On the other hand, microbes taken in by phagocytosis (or endocytosis) are digested and peptides are put onto the cell surface attached to HLA Class II antigens. Cytotoxic T cells are only able to 'see' antigens (peptides) attached to HLA Class I molecules. Since any cell can potentially be infected by a virus, all nucleated cells express these molecules. Helper T cells are only able to recognize microbial antigens (peptides) when they are attached to HLA Class II molecules. Only some cells express these, including macrophages, some dendritic cells and B cells. B cells need help to make antibodies to protein antigens. Pieces of microbial antigens taken into a B cell by its antigen receptor (by endocytosis) appear on the surface attached to HLA Class II to tell T cells that the cell contains microbial antigens and requires help to produce antibodies. Thus whether or not the cell needs to be killed for the sake of the host or 'helped' to remove the microbe from the individual infected cell is determined by which class of HLA molecule the microbial peptide is associated with at the infected cell surface; this, not graft rejection, is the real biological role of the HLA system.

6. On contact with specific microbial antigens, lymphocytes proliferate and develop into clones of effector cells (plasma cells, cytokine-producing cells and cytotoxic cells) and memory cells. The memory cells are long-lived and on encountering the same microbe a second time they respond more rapidly and produce a larger number of both effector and memory cells, leading to a rapid response and further memory. If, as occurs with some carbohydrate antigens, no memory cells are formed, there will be no secondary response and, for example, a vaccine will be ineffective.

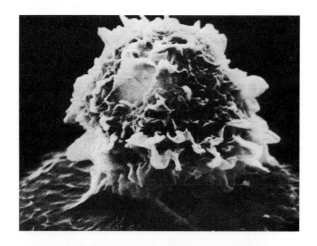

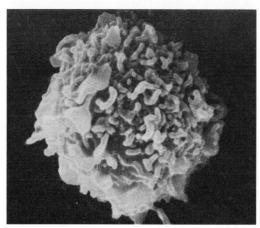

Two of the types of cell that mediate immunity to infection.
Top: *a tissue macrophage, the large phagocyctic cell whose main task is to eat and destroy foreign particles, including bacteria.*
Bottom: *a lymphocyte, whose many functions include the retention of memory of previous infections. In these scanning electron micrographs, the ruffled surface of the cells can be clearly seen; in life these ruffles are in constant motion as the cells move in search of their prey.*

(Reproduced with kind permission from Zucker-Franklin et al 1988 Atlas of blood cells, function and pathology, 2nd edn. Edi Ermes, Milan)

Immunity and infection

6

Case 6.1

On Boxing Day 1899, a 75-year-old man was admitted to a London Hospital complaining of two days' cough, breathlessness, and chest pain. His temperature was 102°F and auscultation with the stethoscope revealed consolidation of one lung, with crackling sounds in the other. He became steadily worse, breathing with difficulty, coughing up blood-stained sputum, and developing a bluish colour. The doctor murmured to the relatives that the outlook was grave, that pneumonia was the 'old man's friend', but that all hope was not lost and New Year's Day would be decisive. Sure enough, on the morning of 1 January 1900, they were amazed to find the patient sitting up and eating a hearty breakfast, and a week later he was home and fully recovered.

Medicine has moved on since 1900, and we now know that this man's pneumonia was probably caused by *Streptococcus pneumoniae*, a Gram-positive diplococcus easily seen by microscopy of the sputum. Nowadays a chest X-ray would have confirmed the consolidation of one or more lobes of the lung, and penicillin or some other antibiotic would have produced a rapid cure. We also know that the sudden improvement on the eighth day of infection was brought about by the antibody response against the bacteria (to be precise, against their capsules) reaching a level sufficient to allow the phagocytic neutrophils crowding the lung alveoli to ingest and destroy them – a perfect example of a life-saving *immune response*. We can take advantage of this knowledge to make a vaccine that will protect most elderly people against this particular infection. Finally, we have learned that it is much commoner and more dangerous in patients who are for any reason deficient in antibody.

Not all infections are dealt with in the same way. If our patient had had tuberculosis, a completely different immune response would have been needed, involving different phagocytes (macrophages) and different lymphocytes (T rather than B). In this chapter we will discuss the main classes of infection and how the immune system copes, or fails to cope, with each. You will see that failure to cope is usually not due to shortcomings on the part of the immune system, but rather to cunning escape strategies by the infectious organisms themselves. Infectious disease is a running battle that has been going on between parasites and their hosts for millions of years, both sides evolving ever more sophisticated weapons without either side completely achieving the upper hand. Unfortunately, despite all our vaccines and antibiotics, the battle looks set to continue for the foreseeable future.

IMMUNITY TO VIRUSES

Viruses pose an interesting challenge to the immune system because they spend the majority of their life inside the cells of the host. The immune system has three answers to this challenge:

1. To prevent the virus getting into a cell, mainly via *antibody*.
2. To make the cell resistant to viral replication, mainly via *interferon*.
3. To kill the cell, complete with the virus inside it, by *cytotoxic T cells* and *natural killer cells*.

Antibody

The most effective blocking factor is antibody against the virus. This can be of any class, since what matters is for the antibody molecule to physically prevent the virus 'docking' with the cell surface receptor (see Chapter 3). Viruses are potent stimulators of both T and B lymphocytes, and specific antibody is found in most virus infections. In the first few days this is mainly IgM, followed by IgG; the IgG1 and IgG3 subclasses are particularly prominent in virus infections. IgA is important in blocking viral entry via the respiratory or intestinal routes. The large, rapid antibody response to a second contact with viruses such as measles is probably responsible for the virtually complete immunity to reinfection.

Antibodies can inhibit viruses in other ways. By activating complement, they can lead to lysis of the viral particle or promote its uptake by phagocytes. Some viruses can even activate complement directly (see alternative pathway, Chapter 5). Antibody bound to a virus-infected cell can lead to its lysis by complement or killing by cytotoxic cells that bear receptors for the Fc portion of the antibody (antibody-dependent cell-mediated cytotoxicity, or ADCC for short). See Figure 6.1 for a summary of these functions of antibody.

One unwelcome effect of antibody is seen with viruses such as dengue which grow in monocytes; IgG antibody against the virus, by promoting

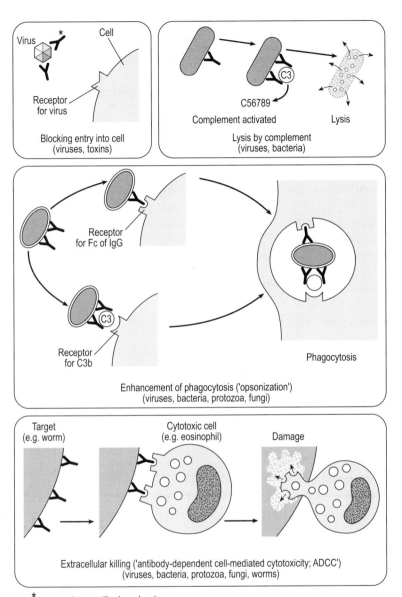

* represents an antibody molecule

Fig. 6.1 Antibody contributes to the elimination of infection in several ways.

attachment to Fc receptors on the monocyte, can actually enhance infection. Other ways in which an antibody response can make the patient worse are considered in Chapter 7 (Immunopathology).

Interferon

Interferon was discovered and given its name because of its ability to interfere with viral replication in cells. The interferons (there are three types,

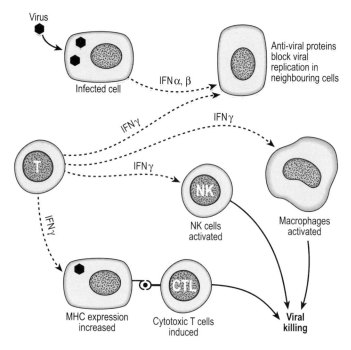

Fig. 6.2 Interferons have numerous antiviral activities.

α, β, and γ) are remarkable molecules in that they attack viruses via several quite separate routes (see Fig. 6.2). They are also interesting in being the first cytokines to be used extensively as therapeutics, against both viral infection and some cancers; the production of interferon α is now a multi-million dollar industry. Finally, it is now clear that many of the symptoms of viral infection (tiredness, muscle pains) are in fact due to overproduction of interferon.

Cytotoxic cells

Two types of cell appear to have evolved mainly to deal with virus infection. They are the natural killer (NK) cell and the cytotoxic T lymphocyte (CTL). Their function is to recognize and destroy virus-infected cells, and though their origins are quite different and they recognize different cell-surface molecules, their methods of destruction are closely similar (see Fig. 6.3). The relative importance of NK cells and CTL in individual diseases is quite hard to assess, but probably NK cells are prominent in the first few days of infection, while CTL, being adaptive cells that require clonal expansion (Chapter 5) play a larger part later and during subsequent infections. For the same reason, CTL activity can be enhanced by vaccination, while that of NK cells cannot. CTL are often referred to as 'CD8' T cells because of the CD8 molecule they carry (Chapter 5).

In addition to viruses, both types of cell may play a role in some bacterial and protozoal infections (and in the rejection of transplants).

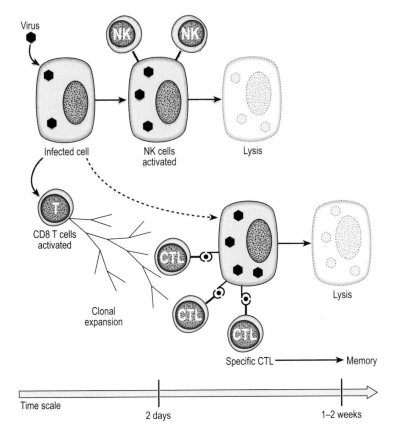

Fig. 6.3 Natural killer and cytotoxic T cells compared.

Escaping immunity

Despite this array of immune defences lined up against them, viruses are very expert at avoiding elimination. As one would expect, their 'escape strategies' are adapted to the host mechanisms listed above. Against antibody and CTL, one of their most effective strategies is to vary their antigens, influenza and HIV being the best-known examples of this. They can also disrupt the function of interferon, and other cytokines too (see Table 6.1). HIV is unusual in that it actually infects T lymphocytes (the CD4 variety) and, by mechanisms not fully understood, leads to their gradual disappearance.

Vaccines

Vaccination started with a virus infection (smallpox) and has had its greatest successes with viruses such as polio, measles, etc. How it works is discussed in Chapter 8.

Table 6.1 Some ways in which infectious organisms evade host defences

Defence mechanism	Evasion strategy	Examples
Mucus + cilia (respiratory tract)	Attach to epithelium Inactivate cilia	*Haemophilus* *B. pertussis*
Gastric acid	Lipid-rich cell wall	*M. tuberculosis*
Bowel movements Diarrhoea	Attach to epithelium	*E. coli*, poliovirus Hookworm
Phagocytosis	Polysaccharide capsule Toxins kill PMN Oxygen radicals inhibited	*Strep. pneumoniae* *Staph. aureus* *Staph. aureus*
Complement	Destroyed by enzymes	*Pseudomonas*
Cytokines	Interferon inhibited Inhibitory cytokines Receptors mimicked	Adenovirus EB virus Pox viruses
Antibody	Fc region blocked Antigenic variation Intracellular habitat	*Staph. aureus* (protein A) Influenza, HIV African trypanosome Viruses, TB
B cells	Polyclonal activation	EB virus
T cells	Infection of T cells Polyclonal activation Deviation of T cells Inhibition of MHC expression	HIV, CMV *Staph.* enterotoxin *M. leprae* Adenovirus
B and T cells	Concealment Uptake of host antigens	Worm cysts Schistosome

Prions

Very little is known about these small peptides, and there is at present no evidence that they induce any useful immunity. A vaccine is therefore, at present, only a remote possibility.

IMMUNITY TO BACTERIA

Extracellular bacteria

Bacteria can be extracellular or intracellular, and immunity against the two types is somewhat different. Extracellular bacteria, such as staphylococci and streptococci, are susceptible to the triad of antibody, complement, and phagocytes, as illustrated by the case of streptococcal pneumonia at the beginning of this chapter, in which the turning point was the production of high levels of IgG against the bacteria, allowing them to be phagocytosed by polymorphonuclear leucocytes (PMN) in the lung (Fig. 6.4). Patients who cannot make IgG antibody, or are seriously deficient in complement, or have defective phagocytes, suffer repeated attacks of this kind of infection (see Chapter 7).

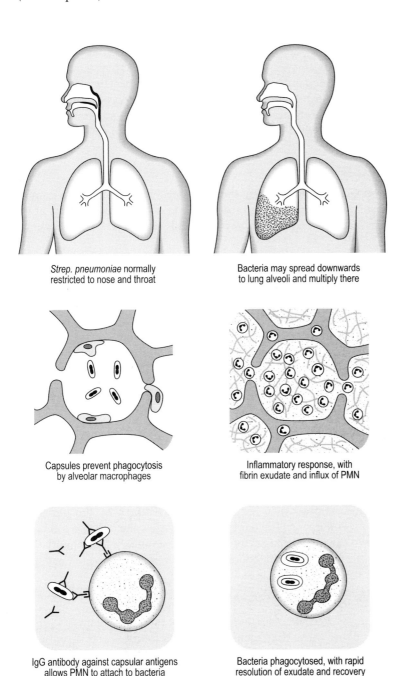

Strep. pneumoniae normally
restricted to nose and throat

Bacteria may spread downwards
to lung alveoli and multiply there

Capsules prevent phagocytosis
by alveolar macrophages

Inflammatory response, with
fibrin exudate and influx of PMN

IgG antibody against capsular antigens
allows PMN to attach to bacteria

Bacteria phagocytosed, with rapid
resolution of exudate and recovery

Fig. 6.4 In bacterial pneumonia, an antibody response is required to enable the bacteria to be phagocytosed. (Each row of diagrams is at a higher level of magnification.)

Escaping phagocytosis

Extracellular bacteria have evolved two very successful defences against the threat of phagocytosis. One is the production of a slimy *capsule* surrounding the bacterial cell, which conceals its surface from the recognition molecules on the phagocyte. Capsules are usually polysaccharide, and their benefit is lost as soon as the host has made antibody against the capsule, because now the phagocyte can recognize the antibody (Fc portion) and engulf the bacterium (see Fig. 6.1). Capsules can also prevent bacteria activating complement via the alternative pathway. The second method is the secretion of *toxins* that kill phagocytes; staphylococci and streptococci are particularly prone to this, which explains their tendency to give rise to pus, which is simply a collection of bacteria and dead phagocytes.

Escaping antibody

Like viruses, bacteria can vary their antigens, but this is not so common as with viruses (Table 6.1). When the variation occurs rapidly – e.g. at weekly intervals – a relapsing pattern of infection is produced (see below).

Intracellular bacteria

Some bacteria, such as the tubercle bacillus, have adapted to survive inside cells, usually macrophages, and these pose a problem somewhat like viruses. Antibody is ineffective, since it would, if anything, facilitate their entry into the macrophage. Fortunately macrophages can switch on a number of powerful killing mechanisms if stimulated by cytokines, particularly interferon-γ. The way in which T lymphocytes detect the presence of intracellular bacteria and then secrete interferon is illustrated in Figure 5.9. This mechanism is usually referred to as *cell-mediated immunity*, and the T lymphocytes involved are the helper subset, often called 'CD4 T cells' (see also Chapter 5).

Escaping intracellular killing

Since macrophages are specialized for killing the microorganisms they engulf, survival obviously requires a counterattack by the parasite. This can take several forms (Table 6.1). In most cases, the balance can be tipped in favour of the macrophages by T cells (see above), which is why the combination of TB and HIV infection is such a deadly one.

Vaccines

Few bacterial vaccines are as successful as those against viruses, the exception being those that act against toxins (tetanus and diphtheria). See Chapter 8 for a description of other bacterial vaccines and some current experimental ideas.

IMMUNITY TO PROTOZOA, FUNGI, AND WORMS

With these advanced eucaryotic parasites, although they induce vigorous immune responses, the resulting immunity is strikingly less successful than against viruses and bacteria. Indeed, there are no cases of complete recovery followed by immunity to reinfection, with the occasional exception of the protozoal skin infection *cutaneous leishmaniasis*. When immunity does develop, as in malaria and schistosomiasis, it can take years and is never more than partial – a situation that suits the parasite, since the patient remains alive to transmit the infection. The usual reason is the very well developed escape mechanisms of the parasite, which include antigenic variation, immunosuppression, and various concealment devices (Table 6.1).

This leads to two unfortunate consequences. First, the likelihood of producing really effective vaccines is considerably reduced. Second, infection tends to be chronic and often lifelong, which means that immune responses continue for much longer than usual, often with harmful effects to the patient (see Immunopathology, Chapter 7). The production of vaccines and chemotherapy against protozoal and worm infections has become a major part of the World Health Organization's programme.

IMMUNITY AND PATTERNS OF INFECTION

Given a knowledge of parasite lifestyle, host immunity, and parasite evasion strategies, one can usually understand the very different courses of different infections. Here are a few examples:

• Short-lived infections lasting a few days (e.g. common virus colds). The symptoms are mainly due to the destruction of epithelial cells in the nose and/or throat. Mucus secretion and sneezing helps to eliminate the virus but also to spread it. Interferon and NK cells are mainly responsible for recovery, antibody being detectable only later. Real immunity never develops because of the enormous number of different viruses and antigenic types ('serotypes').
• Longer infections with recovery after 1–2 weeks (e.g. measles, mumps, streptococcal pneumonia). This is typical of a primary adaptive immune response: antibody or CTL or both. A second infection with the same organism will be eliminated much more quickly and may pass unnoticed – the patient being now 'immune'.
• Repeated attacks of the 'same' infection (e.g. influenza, malaria). These are in fact not exactly the same, but antigenic variants present in the environment.
• Relapsing infection (e.g. brucellosis, relapsing fever, sleeping sickness). Here the antigenic variation is occurring in the patient, often at regular intervals of a week or so.
• Prolonged infection, gradually diminishing over years (e.g. malaria). Despite antigenic variation, effective immunity does eventually develop, possibly because all the possible variants have been encountered.

- Recurrence after many years (e.g. shingles after chickenpox). This is common with herpes viruses, and is due to their ability to 'hide' in the central nervous system.
- Unstable immunity, breaking down if general health declines (e.g. tuberculosis). The balance between bacterial survival strategies and host (cell-mediated) immunity is quite precarious.
- Steadily progressive infection with no sign of immunity (e.g. syphilis, HIV). In the case of HIV, destruction of CD4 T cells prevents effective immunity developing. In the case of syphilis, the organism appears to be resistant to all forms of immune attack.
- Infection with normally harmless organisms. This should make you think of immunodeficiency (see Chapter 7).
- Acute emergencies. Sudden collapse can occasionally be due to infection (e.g. the exotoxin of tetanus or botulism or the endotoxin of Gram-negative septicaemia). A sudden worsening during infection (e.g. with streptococci, meningococci, *E. coli*) may be due to *septicaemia* (organisms in the blood). It is unfortunately the case that some infections, particularly respiratory and urinary, can be acquired in hospital; these are known as *nosocomial*.
- New infections. It should not be forgotten that previously unrecorded infectious organisms do still turn up from time to time. AIDS, legionella, and Lyme disease are three from the last two decades that caused considerable confusion until the cause was identified.

INFECTION AT THE POPULATION LEVEL; EPIDEMICS AND HERD IMMUNITY

When we consider whole populations rather than individuals, some other interesting patterns emerge. Everyone is familiar with the concept of an *epidemic*; it means a sudden increase above the background (or *endemic*) level of infection. Sometimes they are fairly predictable, like the measles and mumps epidemics that occurred every 2–3 years in many countries before vaccines were available. This timing was linked to the school year, since school represents the first contact with large populations in most children's life. There is not an epidemic every year, because in the year following an epidemic the majority of children will be immune, and it takes another year or two to build up a susceptible population large enough to sustain transmission. Thus some children will be spared the disease despite not being immune; this is referred to as *herd immunity*. The same effect can be produced in a population most of whom have been vaccinated (e.g. against diphtheria); the disease virtually dies out and even the unvaccinated are relatively safe from it.

A different pattern is seen with influenza, where epidemics are frequent and irregular, owing to small shifts in the viral antigens, against which nobody is properly immune. Less often a major antigenic change occurs, giving rise to a worldwide outbreak or *pandemic*. It was one of these that killed 20 000 000 exhausted people after World War I. AIDS and (in the

Middle Ages) plague are two other diseases with a pandemic pattern. Note that the science of *epidemiology* is not limited to infectious disease; it covers all diseases (cancer, heart disease, etc.) and all factors that contribute to their incidence.

FURTHER READING

Most books on infectious disease touch on immunity. Here are some that give it more substantial treatment:

Anderson R M, May R M 1991 Infectious diseases of humans. Oxford University Press, Oxford, 757 pp
The mathematical approach to diseases and their spread. Intricate but fascinating.

Giesecke J 1994 Modern infectious disease epidemiology. Arnold, London, 256 pp
Very readable and up to date.

Kreier J P, Mortensen R F 1990 Infection, resistance, and immunity. Harper & Row, New York, 347 pp
Multi-author.

Mims C A, Dimmock N, Nash A, Stephen J 1995 Mims' pathogenesis of infectious disease, 4th edn. Academic Press, London, 414 pp.
A classic in the field for 20 years.

Mims C A, Playfair J H L, Roitt I M, Wakelin D, Williams R 1993 Medical microbiology. Mosby, London, 491 pp
Microbiology and immunology integrated, with copious illustrations and a slide atlas.

Playfair J H L 1995 Infection and immunity. Oxford University Press, Oxford, 154 pp
A short introduction, pitched at second-year undergraduate level.

Tutorial 6

Some more questions to test your knowledge and understanding.

QUESTIONS

1. Compare the roles of B and T cells in viral infection.

2. What factors determine the outcome of the battle between bacteria and phagocytes?

3. What is meant by (a) CTL, (b) NK, (c) PMN, (d) ADCC?

4. Suggest ways in which an infectious organism could vary its antigens.

5. What is herd immunity? Give examples.

6. What would you expect to be the result of being born without a thymus?

ANSWERS

1. The role of B cells is to make antibody, whose main usefulness in viral infection is to block entry of virus into cells. T cells have two main roles: the 'helper' (CD4) type help B cells to make antibody, especially IgG, while the 'cytotoxic' (CD8) ones are responsible for killing cells already harbouring virus. Overall, T cells are probably more critical than B for virus control, since T-cell-deficient babies tend to die of virus infection, while B cell deficiencies predispose to bacterial infection. However, antibody is important in mediating immunity to reinfection with measles, etc.

2. On the bacterial side, capsules, toxins, and the ability to inhibit phagocyte killing mechanisms. On the host side, the availability of antibody and complement to opsonize the bacteria. In turn, bacteria can minimize the effect of antibody by varying their antigens ... and so the battle goes on.

3. CTL are cytotoxic T lymphocytes, the CD8 cells mentioned above. NK cells are natural killer cells, which unlike CTL are not specific for MHC or for individual viruses, and do not develop memory. PMN are the polymorphonuclear leucocytes, also known as neutrophils, which are the first line of phagocytes produced during inflammatory responses and, especially, bacterial and fungal infection. ADCC stands for antibody-dependent cell-mediated cytotoxicity, believed to operate particularly in worm infections.

4. This is an example of a question where you may have to apply intelligent guesswork. In fact, there are three main ways: (a) single *mutations*, such as those responsible for the differences between influenza epidemics, (b) genetic *recombination*, such as when human and animal influenza viruses exchange RNA, to produce a totally new antigenic type, and (c) *gene switching*, where the parasite already has a set of alternative genes and

can switch from one to another. The ever-changing coat proteins of the African trypanosome are made in this way, giving the disease (sleeping sickness) its characteristic relapsing pattern.

5. In herd immunity, a few non-immune individuals are protected by the many immune ones, because the infection finds it difficult to maintain itself without a larger number of 'susceptibles'. It is seen for a year or so after most childhood virus epidemics, and in populations where most people have been vaccinated.

6. The answer to this will be found in Chapter 7, but you should be able to make some predictions, based on what you already know. The thymus makes T cells, so no thymus means no T cells. T cells are vital in virus infection (see above), so no T cells should mean repeated severe virus infections in early childhood. It does – and they are usually fatal, even normally harmless ones such as the attenuated measles vaccine. Immunity to tuberculosis, and to some fungal and protozoal infections, is also drastically impaired, since it depends mainly on cell-mediated immunity.'

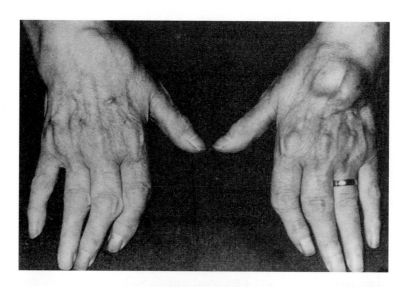

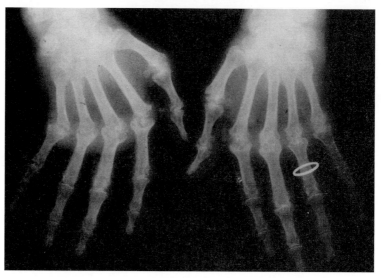

These weak and deformed hands are from a lady with rheumatoid arthritis, and from the X-rays it can be seen that the bones around the metacarpo-phalangeal (knuckle) joints are severely eroded. This damage is due to an attack on the joint by the patient's own immune system – an example of autoimmunity. Unfortunately there are many other autoimmune diseases, and autoimmunity is only one of several ways in which the immune system can harm its possessor, as described in the following chapter.

(Reproduced with kind permission from Dr Michael Shipley, Dept of Rheumatology, UCL Hospital NHS Trust, London.)

Immunopathology and immunodeficiency

7

■ CONTENTS

The immune system, like any other body system, can go wrong. The aggressive lymphoid cells and their products which normally protect us against infectious microorganisms are particularly liable to damage normal cells and tissues. This is what we call *immunopathology* and is mainly the result of overreactivity of the immune system (also known as *hypersensitivity*); it includes the normal rejection of transplants. In contrast, the immune system can be underreactive, with the result that there is an increased susceptibility to infection. We call this *immunodeficiency*. At this point it might be useful to return to Chapter 5 to remind yourself of all the cells and molecules involved in the various types of immune response.

HYPERSENSITIVITY

> **Case 7.1**
> A 12-year-old girl collapsed unconscious in a school classroom a few moments after being stung on her ankle by a bee. Her teacher used an 'epipen' containing epinephrine (adrenaline), which revived her, and the ambulance was called. She was kept in hospital for observation but discharged 5 hours later.

This child is *allergic* to bee stings and she has gone into *anaphylactic shock*. Her collapse is due to a sudden drop in blood pressure as the result of a rapid systemic release of pharmacologically active molecules which cause vasodilation. These molecules, including histamine, are produced by mast cells and basophils (Chapter 5) which have become coated with specific IgE antibodies produced (against an enzyme in the bee's venom, the *allergen*) following a previous bee sting. Note that this will only happen if (1) there has been prior 'sensitization' to the bee venom, and (2) the individual is a 'high producer' of IgE antibody. At the time of her first bee sting she did not have specific antibodies, and would have had no symptoms. The adrenaline in the epipen restored her blood pressure to normal. Sufferers from this kind of allergy who have previously experienced bad reactions to an allergen are advised to carry an epipen.

This type of hypersensitivity reaction is called an 'immediate' or *type 1* hypersensitivity, using the standard classification of hypersensitivities on the basis of the mechanisms of tissue damage suggested by Gell and Coombs (Table 7.1). Note that in many cases the tissue damage is the result of hypersensitivity to relatively harmless non-microbial allergens.

This is the commonest type of hypersensitivity and it has been estimated to occur in around one in five people. Many of you will be allergic to pollen, horse dander or house dust mite. In the latter case it is actually an allergen in the mite's faeces which causes the hypersensitivity! These 'inhalable' allergens can cause hay fever or, more severely, asthma. Other examples of type 1 hypersensitivity are allergies to peanuts and various drugs such as penicillin. The latter have been somewhat reduced in frequency with the increased usage of artificial penicillins. All of these allergens can lead to life-threatening situations as described here. Allergens are generally identified by a skin test in which small amounts of common allergens are injected intradermally – usually on the back of the arm where the skin is relatively thin. If the patient is allergic to one or more of them, within a few minutes the corresponding injection site becomes reddened (weal) and later swollen. Treatment of this type of allergy is generally with sodium chromoglycate which stabilizes mast cells and stops them easily degranulating and releasing their pharmacological mediators; alternatively antihistamines can be used. In severe cases, anti-inflammatory cortico-steroids may be needed. The 'inhalers' used to treat inhaled allergy contain various combinations of these substances.

Case 7.2

At birth, a baby boy (the second child in the family) was seen to be in respiratory distress, with a bluish pallor, and rapidly developed jaundice.
He was immediately given an exchange blood transfusion and within a few days he was discharged home with a healthy complexion and a normal serum bilirubin.

This baby had 'blue baby' syndrome or, as it is technically known, *haemolytic disease of the newborn*. The condition was brought about because his father carried the gene for the red cell surface ('blood group') Rhesus D antigen (Rhesus +ve) whilst his mother was Rhesus –ve. Since these genes are co-dominant the baby had Rhesus D antigen on his red cells. During the pregnancy and especially at the birth of her first child, small numbers of red cells from the baby would have entered the mother's circulation. Because they were Rhesus +ve cells the mother made antibodies to the Rhesus D antigen which she herself did not possess. This would have been of little consequence in the first pregnancy since an insufficient response had been made by the time of birth. However, memory cells with speci-ficity for the Rhesus D antigen were produced and small amounts of

Table 7.1 Classification of hypersensitivities

Hypersensitivity type	Mechanism of tissue damage	Examples of known allergens
Type I 'immediate' (immediate: mins)	Mast cells coated with specific IgE release histamine, etc. Vasodilation, itching, severe form systemic anaphylaxis	Bee/wasp venom, peanut, pollens, house dust mite, drugs (e.g. penicillin)
Type II 'antibody-mediated' (immediate: mins to a few hours)	Antibodies (mainly IgG), with or without complement or cytotoxic cells (ADCC)	Rhesus D antigen, some autoantigens, transplantation antigens
Type III 'immune complex mediated' (intermediate: 4–8 hours)	Antibody/antigen complexes: neutrophils and macrophages are 'activated' to release tissue damaging enzymes, etc. Localized reactions – 'Arthus'; often deposit in kidneys causing damage	Hepatitis B antigen, streptococcal antigens, some autoantigens
Type IV 'delayed-type' (delayed: 24–48 hours)	T-cell-mediated cytokine release	Some metals (e.g. nickel), *M. tuberculosis*, transplantation antigens
Type V 'stimulatory'	'Agonist' effect on hormone receptors	TSH receptor

ADCC: antibody-dependent cellular cytotoxicity; TSH: thyroid stimulating hormone.

antigen passing across the placenta during the second pregnancy were sufficient to produce a large enough IgG antibody response. As you will remember from Chapter 5, IgG from the mother passes across the placenta. In this case the specific anti-Rhesus D antibodies bound to the baby's red cells and they were eliminated as though they were foreign micro-organisms. The severe anaemia can be overcome by 'matched' blood transfusions soon after birth. Most of the specific IgG will have been bound to the erythrocytes and therefore eliminated along with them. The baby will be perfectly capable of making its own red cells from now on. This condition is rarely seen nowadays, being prevented by giving the mother anti-D antibodies after the first delivery, to remove all the Rh+ fetal red cells.

The same *antibody-mediated* or *type II* reaction can occur in individuals receiving blood transfusions for blood loss, anaemia, leukaemia, etc. These 'transfusion reactions' will be considered later when we discuss transplantation of tissues and organs from one individual to another. Other examples of type II hypersensitivity are seen in the case of antibodies made to self cells. These are termed *autoantibodies* and together with transplantation will be dealt with later in this chapter.

Case 7.3

A 12-year-old boy went to his doctor complaining of a sore throat which did not seem to be getting better. He was found to have periorbital oedema (swelling round the eyes), hypertension (raised blood pressure), and proteinuria (protein in his urine), and he was sent for further laboratory tests. Analysis of his blood showed elevated urea and creatinine and raised antibodies to streptolysin O. The doctor prescribed an antibiotic and he was fully recovered 2 weeks later.

This child was suffering from post-streptococcal glomerulonephritis caused by a particular strain of group A haemolytic streptococci. His acute glomerulonephritis and renal failure was due to streptococcal antigen released into the bloodstream forming *immune complexes* with circulating antibodies – a *type III* reaction. Normally, these complexes would be removed by phagocytes, but in this case some were deposited in his kidney, where they fixed complement and attracted neutrophils into the glomeruli. Degranulation of the neutrophils resulted in release of proteolytic enzymes, damaging endothelial and mesangial cells, thus reducing the filtration capacity of the kidney and leading to water retention. Corticosteroids are given to reduce the inflammation and successful treatment with antibiotics should remove the antigen, so no further complexes will be formed. Full recovery is the rule in children, but in older people there may be progression (<10%) to chronic glomerulonephritis and renal failure. Other persistent infectious agents which can cause post-infection kidney damage include Epstein-Barr virus and *Plasmodium* (malaria). Localized deposition of immune complexes can also lead to local inflammatory responses, activation of complement and neutrophil accumulation (e.g. vasculitis) in other organs. The sizes of the immune complexes produced may have a role in whether they deposit in the tissues or kidney. Inhalation of fungi, plant and animal materials can also produce localized reactions by complexing with antibodies at the lung surfaces (farmer's lung and pigeon fancier's lung).

Localized type III responses may be responsible for the reactions to some insect bites, and anyone who has experienced the North American black fly will know how bad these can be! Having been bitten once, the unfortunate individual makes antibodies which then, on a second bite from the fly, form localized immune complexes in the skin, resulting in a severe inflammatory reaction.

Finally, immune complexes can also form when autoantibodies (see later) react with self (auto) antigens. These can also give rise to glomerulonephritis, as happens with the anti-DNA antibodies in systemic lupus erythematosus – appropriately named an 'immune complex disease'.

Case 7.4

During a medical examination for a life insurance policy, a 50-year-old man complained to his GP of severe itching underneath his watch strap which he had noticed for a few weeks. The GP suggested that he leave his watch off for a few days, change the strap, or discontinue using it if the symptoms persisted. He was prescribed a steroid-based ointment for his dermatitis (eczema).

The patient had *contact dermatitis* caused by a small amount of nickel in his watch strap buckle entering his skin through chronic rubbing. Nickel, being a small molecule, had entered his skin and attached to proteins and cells in the dermis. His T cells had become sensitized to this, had recognized it as foreign and produced a cytokine response leading to inflammation. This resulted in a *type IV* hypersensitivity reaction.

Other examples of antigens stimulating this type of skin reaction include dyes, synthetic rubber, chromium, and many plants. It should be stressed that eczema can also be caused by non-immune mechanisms following direct damage to the skin by strong irritants such as phenols, acids, etc. In many cases the aetiology is unknown. Other examples of type IV hypersensitivity are responses to transplantation antigens and to certain microbes where 'granulomas' are produced as the result of chronic inflammation. Granulomas are prominent in patients with tuberculosis and leprosy and are the result of persistence of these microbes inside macrophages and continuous T cell stimulation (see Chapter 2).

The type IV reaction can be used as a skin test to determine whether or not you have been exposed to, for example, tuberculosis in the past. A small amount of mycobacterial antigen is introduced intradermally (Mantoux test). In a positive test, memory T cells accumulate at the injection site and produce cytokines which result in a 'delayed' inflammatory reaction (48–72 hours). Vaccination with BCG is usually recommended if no reaction is evoked.

Case 7.5

A 35-year-old woman complained to her GP of weight loss but increased appetite, excessive sweating and irritability. She had mild tachycardia (rapid heart beat). Her thyroid gland was enlarged and she also had mild exophthalmos (protrusion of her eyes). She was sent for blood tests of thyroid function and an autoantibody screen.

This patient had Graves' disease or thyrotoxicosis resulting from an overactive thyroid. This was caused by autoantibodies (see later section) directed against the thyroid-stimulating hormone (TSH) receptors on her thyroid cells. Production of the thyroid hormones T4 (thyroxine) and T3 is normally regulated by the level of TSH (produced by the pituitary gland) binding to these receptors. In thyrotoxicosis, the autoantibodies bind to these receptors and have the same stimulating effect as the TSH but without the regulatory mechanism. Overstimulation results in raised serum T3 and T4 and failure to control metabolic activity. This 'stimulatory' hypersensitivity is known as *type V*, and like type II is mediated by IgG antibodies. In Graves' disease, myasthenia gravis (where autoantibodies are directed to the acetylcholine receptor), and the blistering skin disease pemphigus, babies born to affected mothers show transient symptoms of the disease due to transmission of the antibodies across the placenta (Chapter 5). These soon disappear owing to the catabolism of the maternal IgG.

In the patients discussed above, the symptoms can, in general, be ascribed to one of the five different hypersensitivity mechanisms. However, there are a number of diseases with an immunological component where more than one type of hypersensitivity is involved in the pathogenesis, e.g. rheumatoid arthritis (see below).

TRANSPLANT REJECTION

Case 7.6

A 55-year-old man with terminal chronic renal failure had been on haemodialysis for 6 months while waiting for a kidney transplant. When a matched donor (from a fatal traffic accident) was found he was given a transplant. Within a few days he had good renal function, but 5 weeks later his renal function began to deteriorate and a renal biopsy taken was shown to contain infiltrating T cells. He was immediately given cyclosporin A and his renal function started to improve. 5 years later he was still alive and well.

Unfortunately, this patient was undergoing *transplant (graft) rejection*. Sometimes the only way of saving a patient's life is to replace diseased tissues or organs with healthy ones from another person (transplantation). Organs and tissues currently transplanted are shown in Table 7.2. Rejection

Table 7.2 Organs and tissues transplanted

Organ/tissue	Main reasons for transplantation
Blood (transfusions)	Severe blood loss, HDN, various anaemias, leukaemias
Kidney	End-stage renal failure
Heart	Heart failure due to infarction, cardiomyopathies, congenital disease
Liver (sometimes with pancreas)	Liver failure
Bone marrow[1]	Stem cell replacement: for immunodeficiencies, metabolic diseases, malignancies
Cornea	Corneal opacity due to trauma, infection
Skin	Burns, major wounds

HDN: haemolytic anaemia of the newborn.
[1]In bone marrow transplantation there is also the problem of the lymphoid cells in the graft producing a response against the recipient's HLA. This 'graft versus host' reaction can be life-threatening but can be reduced/prevented by removal of the lymphoid cells prior to transplantation or treatment of the patient with cyclosporin A.

is due to an immune response made by the recipient against the donor's antigens. The strongest group of antigens to which the immune responses are made are the major histocompatibility molecules – human leucocyte antigens (HLA) – which are important in the normal immune response (Chapter 5). These are the so-called *transplantation antigens*. Like blood groups (discussed below), HLA genes are *polymorphic*, which means that there are many allelic forms in the population as a whole (Table 7.3). Thus each of us carries a different set of these alleles inherited from each parent. These alleles are all expressed as proteins on the surface of the cells of the body

Table 7.3 The human leucocyte antigen (HLA) system

HLA class[1]	Distribution	Genes	Approx. no. of alleles
I	All nucleated cells	A	23
		B	50
		C	10
II	Antigen-presenting cells,	D (DP)	125
	e.g. macrophages,	(DQ)	150
	dendritic cells, B cells	(DR)	60

[1]The HLA genetic locus on chromosome 6 codes for two major classes of glycoprotein molecules, class I and class II; six loci in all. They are co-dominantly expressed at the surface of all nucleated cells (class I) and antigen-presenting cells (class II), i.e. each cell carries 12 different types of molecule. The combinations of these different alleles can run into millions. Class I molecules interact with CD8+ T cells, class II with CD4.

(co-dominantly). Since there are at least six different loci, each with two potentially different alleles, the chance of a donor and recipient having an identical HLA is considerably worse than the chance of winning the national lottery! The mechanisms of graft rejection by the immune system are essentially the same as those responsible for elimination of micro-organisms. In the case described above, the immunopathology is mainly mediated by T cells (essentially type IV hypersensitivity). It is thought that cytokines produced by helper T cells directed to HLA class II antigens and cytotoxic T cells directed against HLA class I antigens are responsible for the rejection, but antibody plays a role too. The rejection was alleviated by cyclosporin A, which works by inhibiting cytokine production by T cells. There are, in fact, several different ways that transplant rejection can be reduced/prevented.

- *Transplantation within families*: Because of the way HLA is inherited, identical twins will accept each other's grafts, and transplants between siblings have a 1 in 4 chance of being accepted.
- *Tissue typing*: The type of HLA class I and class II can be determined in the laboratory and donor and recipient matched accordingly; the better the match, the less the rejection. It is, however, very difficult to match all HLA loci completely.
- *Immunosuppression*: a number of drugs which inhibit immune responses are used, the major ones being corticosteroids, azathioprine and cyclosporin A. These are frequently given as a 'triple' therapy. Note that these drugs act by suppressing the immune response against HLA but will also result in decreased responses to microorganisms – that is, a degree of immunodeficiency.

Antibodies are also made against transplantation antigens and these can be especially pathogenic in the case of kidney and bone marrow grafts. The 'hyper-acute' rejection seen within a few minutes/days of transplantation is due to antibody (type II hypersensitivity). This type of rejection can usually be prevented by 'cross-matching' the donor and recipient, i.e. testing the ability of the recipient's serum to kill (or attach to) the donor's leucocytes. Why should there already be antibodies present to foreign HLA? You will have realized by now that rejection of foreign grafts is mediated mainly through adaptive immune mechanisms, i.e. antibodies and T cells. Thus, when a patient has rejected a graft (e.g. kidney), he will have memory for the foreign HLA on that graft. Before receiving a second graft, it is therefore important to check that that there are no antibodies in the patient which will recognize HLA on the new graft. In addition, pregnant women can be 'sensitized' to paternal HLA on their baby's cells, as a result of mixing of blood during parturition. This can therefore be a problem if they require a transplant later in life.

Blood transfusions

The well-known blood groups are polymorphic antigens on the surface of red cells. In the case of the ABO blood groups, individuals have naturally occurring IgM antibodies to the A or B antigens they do not possess,

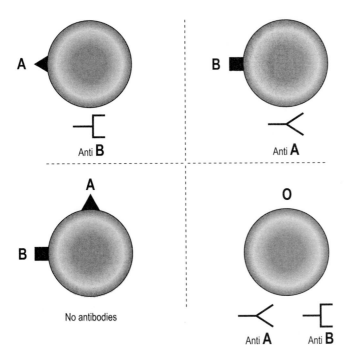

Fig. 7.1 Major blood groups. The major blood group antigens A and B are found on red blood cells. Individuals who are blood group A have natural antibodies to blood group B antigens and vice versa. Individuals with blood group O have neither A nor B on their red blood cells and are therefore *universal donors* since their blood can be given to individuals who are blood group A, B, or AB. Those individuals who are AB do not have antibodies to A or B and therefore are *universal recipients*. Blood group substances are not exclusive to red blood cells and are found in the bloodstream and on the endothelium of kidney blood vessels. Unless matched for the major blood groups, natural antibodies to blood group A or B will attach to the blood group antigens on the blood vessel walls and cause hyper-acute rejection (type II hypersensitivity).

probably through contact with bacteria, etc., which also carry A and B antigens (Fig. 7.1). Occasionally patients are given mismatched blood, which results in a serious 'transfusion reaction' leading to systemic vascular collapse (another example of type II hypersensitivity). This is now, fortunately, relatively rare with the introduction of more stringent blood grouping techniques. It is important to match recipients of kidney and bone marrow grafts for blood groups, since these antigens are also expressed by kidney endothelial cells.

Autografts, allografts, and xenografts

When tissue (e.g. skin) is transplanted from one part of the body to another during plastic surgery, this is an *autograft* and there is no problem of rejection. Grafts from other people are called *allografts*, and have been used for several decades, as described above. Grafts from animals (e.g. pigs' hearts) are known as *xenografts*. They undergo similar rejection to allografts, and there is of course a serious ethical problem as well.

AUTOIMMUNE DISEASES

Case 7.7

A 38-year-old woman told her GP that she was finding it increasingly more difficult to do her embroidery due to stiffness in her fingers and wrist which seemed to be worse in the mornings. She also complained of pains in her knee joints. On examination, she had finger joint swelling and an effusion on one knee. She was put on aspirin and given an appointment with a consultant rheumatologist, who gave her various tests including grip strength and mobility, and X-rays of her joints. Her blood tests showed mild anaemia, a raised erythrocyte sedimentation rate (ESR), increased levels of C-reactive protein (CRP), rheumatoid factors (RF), and raised antinuclear antibodies (ANA). Her X-rays showed mild cartilage degeneration. She was put on indomethacin and an appointment made for 3 months later.

This lady was diagnosed as having rheumatoid arthritis (RA), and you will see a comparison between this and another degenerative joint disease – osteoarthritis – in Chapter 10. The aetiology of RA, three times commoner in women than men, is unknown, but it is very frequently (> 70% of patients) associated with autoantibodies to self IgG, which are therefore known as *rheumatoid factors*. Other autoantibodies found include anti-nuclear antibodies and anti-collagen antibodies. RA is characterized by chronic inflammation of the synovial joints which can lead to cartilage degradation and bony erosions (Fig. 7.2) resulting in joint immobility (for a comparison with *osteoarthritis*, see Chapter 10). The exact pathogenesis of the disease is unclear, but both type IV hypersensitivity and type III (immune complexes) seem to be involved. In the case of the former it is unclear what the autoantigens in the joint are. However, the RA synovial membrane contains many inflammatory cells including T cells, B cells, and macrophages, and there is a high level of the cytokine TNF in the joints, which is associated with the tissue damage. Many plasma cells in the joint can be shown to be making rheumatoid factors. It is likely that the inflammation begins as the result of polymorph infiltration mediated by immune complexes deposited in the joint, which progresses to a chronic form leading to cartilage and bone damage. CRP is an acute phase protein (see Chapter 5) and the level of this in patients with chronic inflammatory diseases is a measure of the amount of inflammation. The ESR reflects the levels of fibrinogen, a component of the clotting pathway which also rises during inflammation.

The presence of autoantibodies designates rheumatoid arthritis as an *autoimmune disease*. In this case the autoantigens include IgG, nuclear antigens and probably collagen. Since these target autoantigens are not exclusive to one organ/tissue we classify this disease as a 'non-organ-specific' autoimmune disease. Autoantigens are also known for some other autoimmune diseases (Table 7.4) and in some cases it is more obvious how the

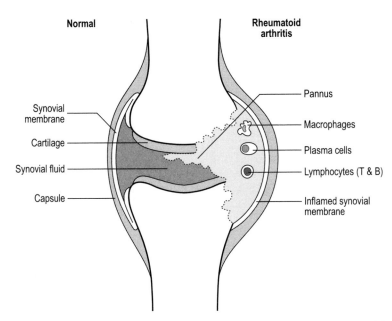

Fig. 7.2 The normal and rheumatoid arthritis joint. The normal synovial membrane (left), surrounded by the joint capsule, contains a few cells which secrete the components of the synovial fluid to lubricate the cartilaginous caps of apposing bones. In rheumatoid arthritis (right), the synovial membrane becomes infiltrated with inflammatory cells including macrophages, T and B lymphocytes, and rheumatoid factor-producing plasma cells. The synovial membrane *migrates* over the cartilage surface as a *pannus* and cells (especially macrophages) produce damaging cytokines (type IV hypersensitivity) which contribute to cartilage degradation and bony erosions. The synovial fluid also contains immune complexes and activated complement components which cause the many neutrophils to release proteolytic enzymes (type II and III hypersensitivity). Unlike osteoarthritis (another degenerative joint disease), RA may involve other tissues, such as heart and lungs. This is always associated with a worse prognosis (see Chapter 10 for a more detailed comparison).

autoantibodies directed to these autoantigens can cause disease. Examples are Graves' disease (see above), where autoantibodies to the TSH receptor result in overactivity of the thyroid, and myasthenia gravis, where auto-antibodies to the acetylcholine receptor block neuromuscular transmission. These are classified as 'organ-specific' autoimmune diseases because the target of the autoimmune reaction is restricted to one organ or tissue. Another example of an organ-specific autoimmune system is given in the next case.

Case 7.8

A 12-year-old girl complained of insatiable thirst and had lost weight over the preceding month. A glucose urine test peformed by her doctor proved positive. Blood tests were carried out and she was found to have hyperglycaemia (raised blood sugar) and further tests revealed that she had autoantibodies to her pancreatic islets of Langerhans cells (ICA). She was diagnosed as having type I diabetes mellitus, juvenile onset, and started on insulin injections.

Table 7.4 Autoimmune diseases

Organ-specific diseases[1]		Non-organ-specific diseases	
Disease	**Autoantigen(s)**	**Disease**	**Autoantigen(s)**
Addison's disease	Adrenal antigens	Ankylosing spondylitis	Vertebral
Autoimmune haemolytic anaemia	Erythrocyte membranes	Chronic active hepatitis	Nuclei, DNA
Graves' disease	TSH receptor	Multiple sclerosis	Brain and white matter
Guillain-Barré syndrome	Peripheral nerves	Primary biliary cirrhosis	Mitochondria
Hashimoto's thyroiditis	Thyroid peroxidase, thyroglobulin	Rheumatoid arthritis	IgG (rheumatoid factor)
Insulin-dependent diabetes mellitus	β cells in pancreas	Scleroderma	Nuclei, lungs, kidney
Myasthenia gravis	Acetylcholine receptor	Sjögren's syndrome	Exocrine glands, kidney, liver, thyroid
Pemphigus	Intercellular matrix	Systemic lupus	DNA, nuclear antigens
Pernicious anaemia	Intrinsic factor	*Several organs affected*	
Polymyositis	Muscle	Goodpasture's syndrome	Basement membrane, kidney, lung
		Polyendocrine organs	Multiple endocrine

[1]*Autoimmune diseases are often classified as organ- or non-organ-specific but there is a great deal of overlap between them. For example, diseases such as Goodpasture's syndrome are classified as organ-specific but affect both kidneys and lung; polyendocrine diseases affect many of the endocrine glands. Note that in many of the non-organ-specific diseases the immune response is directed to intracellular antigens and in particular DNA and other nuclear antigens.*

You will read more about diabetes, and the mechanism by which glucose itself can cause tissue damage, in Chapter 10. Here we are concerned with the fact that it is an organ-specific autoimmune disease since the target of the immune response is the beta (β) cells of the islets of Langerhans in the pancreas which are responsible for producing insulin. How and why the immune system attacks the β cells is unclear. However, it is generally believed that T-cell-mediated (type IV) and autoantibody-mediated (type II) mechanisms contribute to their destruction. There is a genetic predisposition to this disease with a weak association with the DR3 and DR4 alleles at the HLA-DR gene locus (see Table 7.5). In RA there is also a weak association with HLA DR4. Other associations have been found between particular HLA genes and diseases. The strength of these associations is expressed as the *relative risk* (essentially the statistical chance) of a person with a particular HLA allele developing a particular disease. The strongest association is between the B27 allele and ankylosing spondylitis (AS), where there is 90 times more chance of developing AS if you carry the B27 allele. Other risks are less, but still significant.

Despite a lot of knowledge and vigorous research, little is really known about what actually causes autoimmune diseases, although much research effort is being put into it. As indicated in Chapter 5, we are normally tolerant of our own tissues. Breakdown of this 'self-tolerance' leads to development of autoimmunity and autoimmune diseases. Even with the major advances in immunology in recent years, the mechanisms leading to the breakdown of tolerance are poorly understood. It is generally accepted, however, that, at least for some autoimmune diseases, microbial infection may be responsible. Indeed, patients diagnosed with autoimmune diseases often report to their GP that some kind of infection preceded or accompanied the early symptoms. Hormonal changes and genetic factors have also been considered to play a role in autoimmunity.

IMMUNODEFICIENCY

Case 7.9

David, aged 8 months, presented at the casualty department of his local hospital with a painful staphylococcal abscess on his neck. He was given antibiotics and it resolved. At 15 months he had a similar episode and this time he had a surgical incision followed by antibiotics. At 2 years he appeared again at the hospital with two further abscesses. This time he had a high temperature and complained of abdominal discomfort. On physical examination he had a mild hepatomegaly, his blood test showed a high neutrophil count, and a liver scan showed several opaque areas. An NBT test proved positive. His mother pointed out that his brother had died of infection at the age of 3. He was given another course of antibiotics but later developed severe bone infection (osteomyelitis). He was admitted to hospital but the *Staphylococcus aureus* responsible for this infection was resistant to the standard penicillin-like antibiotics (methicillin-resistant *Staph aureus* – MRSA – see Chapter 8) and he died 3 weeks later from overwhelming infection.

Table 7.5 HLA–disease associations

Disease	Locus and associated HLA allele (antigen)			
	A	B	C	DR
Endocrine				
Addison's disease	–	8	–	3(6)
IDDM	–	8(10)[1]	–	3(5), 4(7)
Graves' disease	–	8(2)	–	3(4)
Hashimoto's thyroiditis	–	–	–	5(3)
Rheumatological				
Adult RA	–	–	–	4(7)
AS	–	27(90)	–	–
JAS	–	27(5)	–	–
Reiter's disease	–	27(33)		
Sjögren's syndrome	–	8	–	3(10)
SLE (Caucasian)	–	–	–	2(3), 3(3)
Dermatological				
Psoriasis	–	–	w6(13)	–
Alopecia	–	12	–	–
Behçet's syndrome	–	5(3)	–	–
Pemphigus (AJ)	–	4(25)	–	–
Caucasians	10(3)	–	–	–
Japanese	10(6)	–	–	–
Gastrointestinal				
Ulcerative colitis	–	5	–	–
Atrophic gastritis	–	7	–	–
Coeliac disease	–	8(8)	–	3(11)
CAH	–	8(9)	–	3(14)
Neurological				
Multiple sclerosis	–	7(2)	–	2(5)
Myasthenia gravis	–	8(13)	–	–
Renal				
Goodpasture's syndrome	–	–	–	2(13)
Cancer				
Thyroid	–	–	–	3(3), 1(6)
Allergies				
Ragweed pollen	–	–	–	2(10)

[1] *The relative risk (see text), where known, is shown in parentheses; – no association*
IDDM: insulin-dependent diabetes mellitus; RA: rheumatoid arthritis; AS: ankylosing spondylitis; JAS: juvenile ankylosing spondylitis; SLE: systemic lupus erythematosus; AJ: Ashkenazi Jews; CAH: chronic active hepatitis.

David was diagnosed as having chronic granulomatous disease (CGD), an *immunodeficiency* disease. Immunodeficiency is defined as an increased susceptibility to infection and can be caused in a number of different ways, which are classified as:

- Primary (or congenital) immunodeficiency; an inherent fault in the immune system, usually the result of a genetic defect.
- Secondary (or acquired) immunodeficiency; the result of external factors suppressing the immune system. This might be due, for example, to an insufficient diet (malnutrition) or to direct damage to the immune system, e.g. by HIV.

Normally the immune system goes about its daily task of protecting us against a plethora of infectious organisms. In David's case his neutrophils, although present in normal numbers, lacked the ability to kill ingested microbes. This is a primary immunodeficiency caused by a genetic abnormality resulting in failure in the production of oxygen free radicals when microbes are ingested by neutrophils (see Chapter 5). The NBT (nitroblue tetrazolium) test measures these oxygen free radicals in cells. The opaque areas in his liver were granulomata caused by the inability of the phagocytic cells to deal with the infection (see Chapter 6). Most CGD patients are boys because this is an X-linked disease, but there are some cases which are autosomal (see Chapter 1).

Genetic deficiencies are not restricted to the phagocytic system but can occur in the other three major protection systems – the complement system, the antibody system, and the T-cell-mediated system. The primary immunodeficiency diseases with their defective mechanisms are shown in Table 7.6.

Table 7.6 Primary immunodeficiency

Defence system	Deficiency	Main infections encountered
Phagocytic system	No or reduced numbers of neutrophils; opsonization defects; chemotactic defects; intracellular killing (e.g. CGD)	Extracellular microbes (e.g. *Staph.*, *Strep.*); fungi (e.g. *Candida*); some protozoa and worms
Complement system	Specific complement components Early (e.g. C2, C4, C3) Late (e.g. C6–C9)	Extracellular microbes (e.g. *Staph.*, *Strep.*) Usually fatal *Neisseria*
Cell-mediated immunity	No thymus (DiGeorge syndrome)	Viruses (e.g. CMV, EBV); intracellular microbes (e.g. *Listeria*, TB, *Mycoplasma*); fungi (e.g. *Pneumocystis*); protozoa (e.g. *Giardia*)
Antibody-mediated	No or few B cells (Bruton's agammaglobulinaemia)	Enteroviruses, Echo; extracellular microbes (e.g. *Staph.*, *Strep.*, *Pneumococcus*);
	Lack of response by B cells (common variable deficiencies)	fungi (e.g. *Pneumocystis*); protozoa (e.g. *Giardia*)

It is one thing to identify a defect as being genetic by family studies, etc., but it is another to identify the specific gene abnormality. Nevertheless, several genes have now been identified and mapped to specific chromosomes. This has led to the possibility of replacing a faulty gene with a normal one. Although in its infancy, gene replacement therapy is likely to be the main hope for primary immunodeficiencies in the future. At present, apart from the obvious use of antibiotics, the current therapy is to give bone marrow transplants (containing haemopoietic stem cells), the idea being to reconstitute the recipient with new immune cells carrying the normal gene. Unfortunately there are problems with histocompatibility, as described above.

Case 7.10

A 35-year-old male teacher from Essex had recurrent episodes of perianal herpes over a 2-year period. They were not particularly severe so he had not bothered to get any treatment. However, his most recent recurrence was unusual in that it had lasted 4 weeks and was particularly painful. He decided to go and see if there was any treatment he could get from a sexually transmitted disease (STD) clinic.

After hearing about the herpes the consultant asked about other symptoms and discovered that he had lost weight over the last few months and had noticed that the glands in his armpits became swollen intermittently. He had also noticed that his mouth was very sensitive and complained of occasional severe headaches.

On examination he was seen to have oral thrush (*Candida*) and leucoplakia (white plaques in the mouth). He also had severe and extensive perianal herpes. The consultant felt that advanced HIV disease could explain all these findings. Although the patient had previously been reluctant, he now agreed to have a blood sample taken for HIV antibody testing and CD4 lymphocyte count. He was given oral acyclovir for his herpes and amphotericin lozenges for his oral *Candida*, and cotrimoxazole as prophylaxis against *Pneumocystis*.

When the patient returned to the clinic 3 days later, his HIV antibody test was positive and his CD4 lymphocyte count was 110/mm^3. He was started on triple antiretroviral therapy for HIV (two nucleoside analogues AZT and DDI together with the protease inhibitor Indinovir).

Tests for antibodies to HIV showed that this man was infected with HIV 2 (one of the two common strains of HIV). This was confirmed by identifying genes of the virus in the blood. From his opportunistic infections together with the low CD4+ T cell count, he was diagnosed as having full-blown AIDS (acquired immunodeficiency syndrome).

AIDS is an example of secondary immunodeficiency in which the retrovirus HIV infects and inactivates CD4+ T cells, resulting in progressive immunosuppression. This is thought to be an 'escape' mechanism by which the virus avoids being expelled by the immune system (see Chapter 6 for other ways in which microbes can avoid the immune system). CD4+ T cell counts are normally in the region of 400/mm^3, and below 200 is usually considered to be serious.

Following exposure to HIV, the immune response is similar to that against any virus and an lgM antibody response is made, i.e. the patient becomes 'HIV seropositive' or *seroconverts*. For 2–10 years or more there is a gradual reduction in CD4+ T cells, but the exact mechanism for this is unclear. It appears, at least in part, to be due to CD8+ T cells carrying out their normal function to kill HIV-infected CD4+ T cells (see Chapter 6). Damage to the CD4+ T cells results in severe infections. These can be with normal pathogens but are more often opportunists (see Chapter 4), often fungi such as *Pneumocystis, Candida* ('thrush'), and *Cryptococcus*, viruses such as CMV, HSV, and EBV (see Box 7.1), bacteria (particularly tuberculosis), or the protozoa *Toxoplasma* and *Cryptosporidium*. AIDS patients are also prone to developing tumours, in particular lymphomas such as non-Hodgkin's lymphomas (NHL) and more frequently (up to 10% of patients) Kaposi's sarcoma. The aetiology of these tumours is at present unknown but they do not appear to be due directly to HIV. Treatment is directed towards inhibiting virus replication using nucleoside inhibitors, such as AZT, which block viral nucleic acid synthesis, and protease inhibitors, which specifically block synthesis of new HIV proteins. The new triple therapy as given to the above patient has shown great promise in the early stages following seroconversion.

Box 7.1 lists the other main causes of secondary immunodeficiency. In the Western world, probably the most frequent is the use of *drugs* (chemotherapy) and *radiation* (radiotherapy) for cancers (see Chapter 12). These target the rapidly dividing cells of a tumour but may also inhibit production of new blood cells from the bone marrow. Neutrophils and platelets, because of their short lifespan (a few days), are the first to suffer, resulting in neutropenia and thrombocytopenia. Patients receiving these therapies are checked regularly for 'bone marrow depression' by blood count and, if needed, bone marrow biopsy.

Worldwide, however, the commonest cause of immunodeficiency is *malnutrition*. All cells require nutrients for normal function (see Chapter 1) in the form of proteins – as a source of amino acids – energy-giving carbohydrates and fats, vitamins and various trace elements which are important for aiding the efficiency of enzymes. Deficiencies in these nutrients can affect normal cell function, and cells of the immune system are no exception. In countries where famines are frequent, protein-calorie malnutrition is a real problem and can give rise to severe immunodeficiency.

Patients with uncontrolled diabetes can be susceptible to certain kinds of bacterial infection, mainly due to impaired neutrophil function, and poor peripheral circulation can further lead to infected ulceration, e.g. in the lower limbs. Staphylococci, pneumococci, and *Candida* are the commonest infections. As people get older they tend to experience more infections. The overall bulk of the lymphoid tissue decreases with age and the functions of several components of the immune system are thought to be reduced with age, including phagocytes, NK cells, and T cells (see Chapter 13).

■ **BOX 7.1 Causes of secondary immunodeficiency**

- Malnutrition (protein and/or calorie deficiency, iron, zinc).[1]
- Trauma; burns; area exposed to microbes and loss of antibodies; surgery, splenectomy.
- Some cancers of the immune system, e.g. lymphomas (Hodgkin's, NHL), leukaemias (CLL and myelomas). Cancers of some other systems, e.g. liver tumours.[2]
- Cytotoxic/cytostatic drugs used to treat cancers and autoimmune diseases, and to prevent transplant rejection (chemotherapy), e.g. cyclophosphamide, steroids, and irradiation (radiotherapy).
- Loss of immune cells and/or antibodies from the body, e.g. nephrotic syndrome[3] and lymphangiectasia.[4]
- Infectious agents: HIV, CMV, EBV, malaria parasite (*Plasmodium*).[5]
- Other diseases, e.g. diabetes mellitus.[6]
- Ageing.[6]

NHL: non-Hodgkin's lymphoma; CLL: chronic lymphocytic leukaemia; HIV: human immunodeficiency virus; CMV: cytomegalovirus; EBV: Epstein-Barr virus.
[1]*Widely seen in countries where famines are common.*
[2]*See Chapter 12 for details of tumours.*
[3]*This results in a change in the kidney filtration, leading to proteinuria which includes antibodies as well as other small proteins.*
[4]*Lymphangiectasia results in loss of lymphocytes into the intestine.*
[5]*The mechanism by which the malaria parasite produces immunosuppression is unknown but may alter the important cytokine network (Chapter 5).*
[6]*Patients with diabetes and old people tend to have increased numbers of infections (see text).*

The reduced ciliary function in the bronchus as the result of thick mucus accumulation in cystic fibrosis (see Chapter 1) or of heavy smoking predisposes to bronchial infections. Similarly, blockage of tear ducts resulting in reduced tear flow can lead to eye infections. There are also conditions, not well understood, in which the antibacterial secretions of the skin seem to be the only defect; this is not strictly speaking 'immunodeficiency', but it results in intractable skin infections.

FURTHER READING

Gupta S, Griscelli C (eds) 1993 New concepts in immunodeficiency diseases. Wiley, Chichester, 503 pp

Isenberg D, Morrow J 1995 Friendly fire: explaining autoimmune disease. Oxford Medical Publications

Krentz A J 1997 Diabetes (colour guide). Churchill Livingstone, Edinburgh, 91 pp

Life, death and the immune system. Scientific American (special issue), September 1993

Mygind N, Dahl R, Pedersen S, Thestrup-Pedersen K 1996 Essential allergy. Blackwell Science, Oxford, 430 pp

Shipley M 1993 A colour atlas of rheumatology, 3rd edn. Wolfe, London, 175 pp

Stites D P, Terr A I, Parslow T G 1994 Basic and clinical immunology, 8th edn. Prentice-Hall, Englewood Cliffs, NJ
A good book covering basic immunopathology.

Tutorial 7

QUESTIONS

1. Why is it necessary to immunosuppress patients receiving kidney grafts?

2. Give three examples of primary and three examples of secondary immunodeficiency.

3. What do you think is the difference between autoimmunity and autoimmune disease?

4. What can be learned by the use of skin testing?

5. What is an immune complex and how could it cause disease?

ANSWERS

1. Tissues or organs transplanted from one person to another are normally rejected because of histocompatibility antigens. The polymorphic molecules (see Table 7.3) are a strong stimulus for the recipient's immune system. To reduce rejection of the kidney graft, it is best (if possible) to use family members as donors. Because the histocompatibility genes are usually inherited en bloc, siblings will inherit half of the HLA genes from each parent and siblings will thus be HLA identical 1 in 4 times. In large families, therefore, a graft can often be found that is completely matched for HLA. But if an appropriate relative is not available, tissue typing will be needed to identify HLA of both donor and recipient. Reducing the number of different HLA alleles between donor and recipient will reduce the magnitude of the rejection process, but will not altogether prevent it. In most cases, therefore, it is necessary to give immunosuppressive drugs to reduce the immune response against the donor HLA.

2. *Primary (congenital, genetic) immunodeficiencies*: Chronic granulomatous disease: the phagocytic cells of the child (usually a boy) fail to kill phagocytosed microbes, leading to the formation of immune granulomata in many organs (Case 7.9). DiGeorge syndrome: the lack of a thymus resulting in no T lymphocytes being produced. The patient suffers from viral and some fungal infections. Bruton's disease or agammaglobulinaemia: a disease in which the patient lacks antibodies. No B lymphocytes are found in the circulation and no plasma cells in the lymphoid tissues. A gene controlling 'activation' of B cells has been shown to be abnormal in these patients. *Secondary (acquired) immunodeficiencies*: Malnutrition is the most serious cause worldwide. Proteins (amino acids for building proteins, e.g. antibodies) and carbohydrates (for calories), together with iron, copper, vitamins, and the trace elements (see Chapter 1), are all necessary for health. Reduction of intake in these can lead to severe infections and death. Childhood infections such as chickenpox and measles, not usually life-threatening to children receiving a normal diet, are a major cause of death to children in famine-bound countries. HIV causes immunosuppression (acquired immune deficiency syndrome) by infecting helper T lympho-cytes via CD4 on their cell surface. This results in malfunction of this important cell, which normally helps most of the cells of the immune response to carry out their function, i.e. macrophages, cytotoxic T cells, B cells, NK cells. Cytotoxic drugs and radiation used in cancer therapy are a common cause of immunosuppression in developed countries.

3. *Autoimmunity* is anti-self reactivity which may or may not lead to *autoimmune disease* (i.e. pathology). The job of cytotoxic T cells is to kill self cells infected with viruses, etc. This is one example of beneficial auto-reactivity. Patients can have autoantibodies even though they do not have an autoimmune disease. For example, patients infected with Epstein-Barr virus (glandular fever) often have antibodies to DNA and to antibodies themselves (RF – see Case 7.7), but these are not normally pathogenic. Patients with malaria also have anti-DNA antibodies. It is quite common for old people to have a variety of non-pathogenic autoantibodies. When autoantibodies are pathogenic this leads to autoimmune disease – for example, autoantibodies to the acetylcholine receptor in myasthenia gravis or the TSH receptor in thyrotoxicosis. The presence of autoantibodies following infection gives us a clue that microbes are important in the aetiology of autoimmune diseases.

4. Skin tests are used by clinical immunologists to identify the antigen(s) and mechanisms involved in a suspected hypersensitivity reaction. The principal ones are (1) the immediate test for type I (allergic) hypersensi-tivity, read 10 minutes later, (2) the patch test for contact sensitivity, and (3) the Mantoux and related intradermal tests for exposure to tuberculosis and some other intracellular parasites. The latter two tests both measure type IV (T-cell-mediated) hypersensitivity and are read 2–3 days later.

5. An immune complex is formed whenever antibody binds to antigen. If several antibodies bind to several molecules of antigen, a large complex will result, which would normally be removed by cells of the mononuclear phagocyte system (see Chapter 5). Once the responsible antigens are eliminated, specific antibody levels drop. However, when antigens are not effectively removed (e.g. chronic infections), immune complexes can be trapped in various sites, notably the kidney, which is where blood is filtered. Alternatively they may attach to endothelial cells of the blood vessels, leading to vasculitis. The attached immune complexes activate complement components which in turn activate neutrophils. These, unable to phagocytose the tissue to which the immune complexes are attached, release toxic materials and proteolytic enzymes, together with cytokines which further increase the accumulation of immune cells in the site (type III hypersensitivity). *Autoantigens* are, by definition, persistent antigens, since they are derived from 'self' and can never be eliminated. Thus immune complexes formed with autoantigens (e.g. DNA) often lead to type III hypersensitivity reactions and tissue damage. Diseases caused in this way are often referred to as 'immune complex diseases', examples being systemic lupus erythematosus and rheumatoid arthritis.

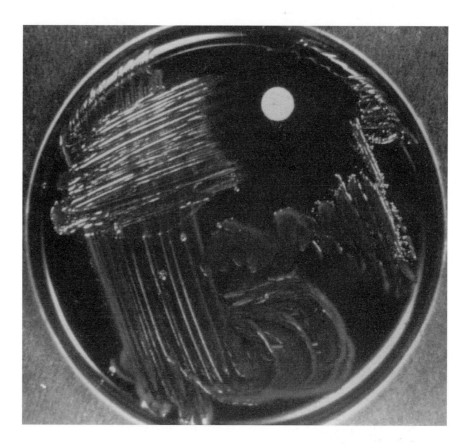

In this culture on blood agar from a suspected urinary infection, there is a heavy growth of Escherichia coli ('E. coli'). The small white disc contains the antibiotic trimethoprim, and the bacterial growth is clearly inhibited around it, showing that the organism is sensitive to this drug, which would therefore be appropriate for treatment. In this chapter we discuss the use of drugs to treat infection and of vaccines to prevent it.

(Reproduced with kind permission from Dr J. Holton, UCL Medical School, London.)

Controlling infection

8

■ CONTENTS

In Chapter 3, we described the case of Dr Petrie, who caught malaria on a trip to India, and on his return was fortunately diagnosed and cured. But what about the millions of Indians, Africans, and other dwellers in the tropics who are regularly exposed to malaria, and of whom some 2 million, mostly children, die every year? And what about those other major killers tuberculosis, infantile diarrhoea, and respiratory infections? Given a limited budget, what is the best approach? This is the problem that faces health authorities all over the world, and particularly the World Health Organization, which raises money from member states and, guided by experts, is responsible for deciding how it should be spent.

The solution, in theory, is simple: either prevent contact between the patient and the parasite, or do something to eliminate the parasite from the patient. In practice, the control of infection falls into four categories:

1. *Public health* measures to minimize exposure of individuals to infectious organisms.
2. *Vaccination* ('active immunization') to induce the patient's immune system to eliminate the infectious organism, or prevent the damage it causes.
3. *Passive immunization*, to confer on the patient the benefit of immunity raised in some other individual or animal.
4. *Chemotherapy* – the use of drugs to kill the infectious organism without harming the patient.

In this chapter, we shall look at all four strategies, comparing their strengths and weaknesses.

PUBLIC HEALTH MEASURES

This is a huge subject, which cannot be fully covered in a short chapter. Many health measures are fairly obvious, but they are often difficult to put into practice. They can usefully be divided into those that operate in the community as a whole, and those unique to the hospital environment.

Infection in the community

If Dr Petrie had slept in a mosquito net, he would not have got malaria. If we all wore masks as soon as we caught a cold, colds would not spread. If you wash your hands and drink only bottled water, you should avoid traveller's diarrhoea. When the pump in Broad Street was closed down in 1855, cholera disappeared from that part of London. Rich Brazilians, who do not live in slums infected with the bugs that carry *Trypanosoma cruzi*, do not get Chagas' disease. And so on. Clearly in a perfect world there would be a lot less infection!

About 30 infectious diseases are *notifiable*, which means that the medical profession has a duty to report every case to the local health authority so that contacts can be monitored (Box 8.1). For those who work with infectious organisms, they are classified into *categories*, depending on the likelihood and severity of disease and of its spread, and the availability of treatment. For example, HIV and TB are Category 3, and the deadly Marburg and Ebola viruses are Category 4 (see Appendix 2 for a fuller list).

■ **BOX 8.1 Some infectious diseases have to be notified by the doctor to the Health Authority so that contacts can be traced**

Anthrax	Meningitis	Smallpox
Cholera	Meningococcal infection	Tetanus
Diphtheria	Mumps	Tuberculosis
Dysentery	Ophthalmia neonatorum	Typhoid
Encephalitis	Paratyphoid	Typhus
Leprosy	Plague	Viral haemorrhagic fevers
Leptospirosis	Rabies	Viral hepatitis
Malaria	Relapsing fever	Whooping cough
Measles	Scarlet fever	Yellow fever

In addition, there are some occupation-related diseases which it is the employer's duty to report. These include:

Brucellosis	Leptospirosis
Psittacosis	Lyme disease
Legionellosis	Q fever

Infection in hospitals

The idea that a patient can catch an infectious disease in hospital offends many people, but it is unfortunately all too true. Such infections are known as nosocomial (from Latin *nosocomium* hospital), and they can be very serious because hospital patients are often more than usually susceptible to infection as a result of injuries, surgery, or debilitating illness. Some are brought in by the patients themselves, but more often they are picked up from staff or from the ward environment, including equipment. The latter two sources can be particularly dangerous, because the organisms have a high probability of being resistant to common antibiotics. The best-known example is the methicillin-resistant *Staph. aureus* (MRSA) carried on the skin and in the nose of many healthy people, but *Streptococcus pyogenes*, *E. coli*, *Pseudomonas*, and *Candida* are also major problems. Overall, the sites most commonly affected are wounds, the urine, and the respiratory system.

Sterilization

An important part of controlling hospital infection is the sterilization and disinfection of contaminated material. Sterilization implies the inactivation of all microbes, including bacterial and fungal spores. Surgical equipment is sterilized by autoclaving with steam at a temperature of 121°C and under a pressure of 15 lb/in². Heat-sensitive equipment is sterilized by ethylene oxide, and solutions by filtration through 22 μm pores, which filter out microbes. Radiation in the form of X-rays and ultraviolet (UV) light is also used, e.g. for surgical gloves, acting mainly on microbial DNA by the creation of thymine dimers and/or free radicals.

Disinfectants kill most microbes but not all (e.g. bacterial spores). They are mainly chemicals which act:

- by disrupting cell membranes (alcohol, detergents, phenol);
- by modifying proteins (chlorine, formaldehyde/glutaraldehyde, acids, alkalis, heavy metals). Chemicals that can safely be used on the skin and mucous membranes are termed antiseptics (ethanol, hydrogen peroxide, iodine);
- by modifying nucleic acids (gentian violet).

VACCINATION

In Chapter 5, we quoted Pasteur's famous experiment with rabies vaccination, mentioning how it was preceded by Jenner's work with smallpox, and followed by vaccines against tetanus, diphtheria, and many common virus infections. Today it is common practice worldwide to vaccinate against the diseases listed in Table 8.1, though there are some variations depending on local conditions.

The rationale of vaccination is simple: the infectious organism in a harmless form, or an antigen derived from it, is introduced into the patient, usually by injection but sometimes by mouth. B and/or T lymphocytes recognize it and mount a primary response, giving rise to *memory cells*. Subsequent contact with the fully infectious organism will now stimulate a *secondary* response, with all its advantages of speed, size, and duration (see Chapter 5). Thus the essential requirements for a good vaccine are a safe antigen that stimulates the right lymphocytes. To achieve this, different types of preparation are used for different diseases (Table 8.1).

Table 8.1 Vaccines are available for many, but not all, infections

When given	Disease	Type of vaccine	Comments
Vaccines in general use			
2, 3 and 4 months	Diphtheria	Toxoid	IM or SC
	Tetanus	Toxoid	with alum
	Whooping cough	Killed bacteria	adjuvant
	Polio	Attenuated virus[1]	Oral
	Haemophilus B	Capsular polysac.	IM or SC
12–18 months	Measles	Attenuated virus	IM
	Mumps	Attenuated virus	IM
	Rubella	Attenuated virus	IM
5 years	Diphtheria		Boost,
	Tetanus		as above
	Polio		
10–14 years	BCG[2]	Attenuated tubercle bacillus	
Leaving school	Tetanus		Boost,
	Polio		as above
Vaccines for those at risk			
Hospital staff	Hepatitis B	Surface antigen	3 doses
Travel	Typhoid; cholera	Killed bacteria	
Travel	Yellow fever	Attenuated virus	
Travel	Hepatitis A		
Elderly	Influenza	Killed virus	Also nurses, etc.
Elderly	Pneumococcus	Capsular polysac.	
Epidemics	Meningococcus	Capsular polysac.	
Post-exposure	Rabies	Killed virus	
Vaccines not available or experimental			
Adenovirus, rhinovirus, herpes viruses, RSV, HIV, staphylococci, streptococci, gonococcus, *E. coli*, syphilis, all fungi, protozoa,[3] worms			

IM: intramuscular; SC: subcutaneous.
[1] *There is also a killed polio vaccine (Salk).*
[2] *In tropical countries, where TB is common, BCG is given at birth.*
[3] *There have been several moderately successful trials of malaria vaccines.*

Living and non-living vaccines

The first vaccine, vaccinia (cowpox), was a normal living animal virus. Unfortunately no other animal viruses have been found to be both effective and safe, so most viral vaccines are made by *attenuating* the human virus. This is done by making the virus genome mutate, by forcing it to grow in non-ideal conditions. Mutants are repeatedly screened for antigenicity and virulence (in animals!) until one is found that has retained antigenicity but lost virulence. Yellow fever, and the common childhood viruses measles, mumps, and rubella, are successful examples.

Sometimes it proves impossible to make stable and effective attenuated viruses, and then it is necessary to use *killed* viruses. At present, the vaccines against rabies and influenza are of this type. Polio is unusual in that there are both attenuated (Sabin) and killed (Salk) vaccines on the market. In one case it has been possible to produce a particular virus protein by recombinant DNA technology; this is the extremely successful hepatitis B surface antigen.

With bacteria, the situation is rather different. The two most effective vaccines are those against the exotoxins of tetanus and diphtheria. Only one attenuated vaccine has stood the test of time: the BCG (bacille Calmette-Guérin) vaccine against tuberculosis, and even this varies widely in its effectiveness in different populations. The remaining bacterial vaccines are mostly whole killed organisms, but there is one special group of capsulated organisms (meningococcus, pneumococcus, *Haemophilus*) where the capsular polysaccharides make good vaccines, though they sometimes need coupling to proteins to enable them to induce proper memory.

Protozoa, fungi, and worms remain a major problem, since there is no successful vaccine against any of them. Vaccines against malaria, leishmaniasis, and schistosomiasis are at present in the experimental/field trial stage.

Safety and limitations

Vaccination is the only medical treatment imposed on perfectly healthy individuals. Therefore safety is absolutely vital. Table 8.2 lists the main safety considerations, of which three are worth further comment.

Living attenuated organisms are a serious risk for two reasons. Firstly, being produced by a process of random mutation, they can theoretically revert to the normal virulent ('wild') type, and this has in fact occurred with the attenuated (oral) polio strains, in one case causing a small outbreak of paralytic polio. The answer is to produce strains with more mutations, and this is nowadays done with help from molecular biologists rather than by the original 'hit or miss' method.

The second danger with attenuated organisms is that they can cause serious disease in immunodeficient patients. Indeed there have been deaths from vaccinia, BCG, and measles vaccines in such patients. The general rule, therefore, is that only non-living vaccines are used, though obviously there will be cases where the danger from the vaccine may be outweighed by the danger from the infection; for example, children with leukaemia are often given the attenuated VZV (chickenpox) vaccine.

Table 8.2 Safety is a key issue with vaccination

Type of vaccine	Problem	Examples
Living attenuated	Reversion to wild type	Polio (Sabin), especially types 1 and 2
	Severe disease in immunodeficient patient	Vaccinia, BCG, in T cell deficiency
	Instability (need for unbroken 'cold chain')	Attenuated viruses
Killed	Poor immunity Need for adjuvant[1] Need for boosts	Meningococcus type B Tetanus Diphtheria

All	Toxic components
	    Bacterial endotoxins
	    Egg proteins
	Incomplete killing (rare)
		
		B. pertussis
		Attenuated viruses

[1] *The most widely used adjuvant is alum (aluminium hydroxide), which enhances the effect of the vaccine.*

The third point concerns side-effects. Vaccines can contain impurities, due either to errors in production or to unavoidable components of the vaccine. Two well-known examples are hypersensitivity to the minute amounts of egg protein that may contaminate viruses grown in eggs, and the (still controversial) effect of the *Bordetella pertussis* (whooping cough) vaccine in causing fits and brain damage in children. The fear of expensive litigation is one of the factors that has discouraged many biopharmaceutical firms from getting involved in vaccine development.

Taking all these risks together with the fact that very few vaccines are absolutely guaranteed to protect 100% of people (the highly successful hepatitis B vaccine protects about 95%), you will see that vaccination is a procedure to be undertaken with forethought and care. Nevertheless, it remains probably the most cost-effective method ever invented for improving the health of the human race. It has eliminated smallpox, and, if vigorously applied, may eliminate polio, measles, mumps, and rubella within the next generation, and none of this could have been achieved by other means.

PASSIVE IMMUNIZATION

You will recall the tetanus antitoxin that saved so many lives in World War I (see Chapter 4). This principle of injecting preformed antibody, or *antiserum*, into a patient is referred to as passive immunization, and though much less common nowadays, is still used in certain emergency situations, generally where the patient has already been exposed and there is not time for him to mount an effective response to a vaccine (Table 8.3). One unusual disease is rabies, where the incubation period is so long – about 6 weeks –

Table 8.3 Passive immunization is used in some emergencies

Indication	Preparation used	Examples
Post-exposure	Immune human serum	Tetanus Rabies (with vaccine) Chickenpox[1] Measles Hepatitis A Hepatitis B
	Immune horse serum	Diphtheria Gas gangrene Botulism Bite of snakes, spiders, etc.
Prophylactic	Pooled human serum	Hepatitis A (e.g. pre-travel) Hypogammaglobulinaemia[2] Some autoimmune diseases[2]
	Anti-Rhesus D serum	Rhesus incompatibility[3]

[1] *In newborn or immunodeficient children.*
[2] *See Chapter 7.*
[3] *This prevents sensitization of RhD– mothers by RhD+ babies.*

that there *is* time for this, so patients bitten by rabid animals are given both the normal vaccine (to induce an immune response) and an injection of antiserum (to mop up any virus that has not yet entered the nerves via which the virus travels to the brain). An exotic condition where passive immunization is the only treatment is snakebite, and here the antiserum is known as *antivenom*.

The injection of pooled normal human immunoglobulins to protect patients with antibody deficiencies was discussed in Chapter 7, but it is in fact only a special example of passive immunization.

CHEMOTHERAPY

A generation after Pasteur, the great German chemist Paul Ehrlich introduced the concept that drugs might be made that killed infectious organisms without damaging their host – the principle of *chemotherapy*. Then Sir Alexander Fleming discovered that such compounds were actually made by microorganisms themselves – the *antibiotic* penicillin being the first example of this. Today the production of new antibiotics and chemotherapeutics is a multibillion dollar industry, with an estimated 300 new products per year. Since chemotherapy (the term is nowadays used to include antibiotics) has had its main impact on bacterial infections, we will consider these first.

Antibacterial therapy

The success of penicillin is due to the fact that bacterial cell walls are made by a completely different process from mammalian ones, and beta-lactams (the group of chemicals to which penicillin belongs) can interfere with this. Other antibacterials act against bacterial nucleic acid and protein synthesis, and there are some whose action is not fully understood. Table 8.4 lists the ones you are most likely to come across.

There are two major problems with chemotherapy: toxicity and resistance. Toxicity is the more serious, and has been responsible for hundreds of drugs not passing today's very strict safety tests, and for several being withdrawn later. It can occur at three levels: (1) a direct effect on some vital body component, e.g. streptomycin on the auditory nerve or chloramphenicol on the bone marrow; (2) by eliminating one organism it may leave the field open for others, e.g. tetracycline on the intestinal flora; and (3) the immune system may react against the drug to produce a hypersensitivity (see Table 8.5 and Chapter 7); penicillin is one of the main culprits here.

Resistance is due to the microorganism mutating a gene or genes to avoid the antibiotic (see Table 8.6). Unfortunately bacteria, with their rapid

Table 8.4 The antibacterial drugs in common use

Drug	Action	Examples of clinical use
Beta-lactams	Inhibit cell wall	Gram^{+ve} infections
Penicillins	peptidoglycan synthesis	Pneumonia, meningitis
(Flu)cloxacillin	"	Bone and joint
Ampicillin	"	Many
Cephalosporins	"	Gram^{-ve} infections
Cefotaxime	"	Gram^{-ve} infections
Ceftazidime	"	Gram^{-ve} infections, esp. *Pseudomonas*
Vancomycin	"	Penicillin-resistant *Staph.*
Aminoglycosides	Inhibit protein synthesis	Gram^{-ve} infections
Gentamycin	"	Gram^{-ve} infections
Streptomycin	"	Tuberculosis
Tetracyclines	"	Chlamydiae, Rickettsiae
Chloramphenicol	"	Chlamydiae, Rickettsiae
Erythromycin	"	Many, esp. Gram^{+ve}
Clindamycin	"	Gram^{+ve} and $^{-ve}$
Sulphonamides	Inhibit nucleic acid synthesis	Gram^{-ve}, esp. urine
Trimethoprim	"	Gram^{-ve}, esp. urine
Rifampicin	"	Tuberculosis
Metronidazole[1]	"	Anaerobic bacteria
Ethambutol	"	Tuberculosis
Isoniazid	Inhibit mycolic acid synthesis	Tuberculosis

[1]*Also active against protozoa (see Table 8.8).*

Table 8.5 Some unwanted side-effects of commonly used antimicrobial drugs

Drug	Mechanism	Clinical effect
Antibacterial		
Penicillins	Hypersensitivity	Anaphylaxis (about 1 in 10 000)
		Haemolytic anaemia
		Skin rashes (up to 1 in 4)
	Fits, spasms	High-dose benzylpenicillin only
Aminoglycosides	Kidney damage	Renal failure
	Auditory nerve damage	Dizziness, deafness
Tetracyclines	Altered gut flora	Diarrhoea
	Staining of growing teeth	Children under 9
Chloramphenicol	Bone marrow failure	Pancytopenia
		Aplastic anaemia (1 in 30 000)
Erythromycin		Nausea, vomiting (rare)
Sulphonamides	Hypersensitivity	Skin rashes
Trimethoprim	Bone marrow suppression	Neutropenia
Rifampicin		Skin rashes, jaundice (4%)
Metronidazole		Peripheral neuropathy
Isoniazid		Jaundice (1%), convulsions[1]
Antiviral (see also Table 8.7)		
Zidovudine (AZT)	Bone marrow damage	Anaemia, leucopenia
Interferons		'Flu-like' symptoms
Other (see also Table 8.8)		
Amphotericin B (antifungal)		Renal damage
Ketoconazole (antifungal)		Nausea, vomiting
Quinine (antimalarial)		Cardiac arrhythmias, ear, eye[1]

Leucopenia: low white blood cell count; pancytopenia: all blood cells low.
[1]Only with overdosage.

reproductive rate, can evolve resistance quite fast, and many antibiotics have become almost useless within 5–10 years of their introduction. The classic example is *Staphylococcus aureus*, now widely resistant to penicillin, which it achieves by producing an enzyme, beta-lactamase, that destroys the drug. A synthetic penicillin derivative, methicillin, has been manufactured which resists this enzyme, but some staphylococci have also developed resistance to this. They are known as methicillin-resistant *Staphylococcus aureus* (MRSA) and are one of the most feared hospital infections. A new antibiotic, mupyrocin, offers the best hope.

Table 8.6 Resistance to commonly used antimicrobial drugs

Drug	Mechanism	Comments
Antibacterial		
Penicillins	Production of beta-lactamase New penicillin-binding proteins Reduced membrane permeability	Common (Gram^{+ve} and $^{-ve}$) MRSA only Gram $^{-ve}$
Aminoglycosides Tetracyclines Chloramphenicol Sulphonamides	Induction of enzymes that inactivate the antibiotic	Frequently occur together because genes carried on same plasmid
Tetracyclines	Drug pumped out?	
Suphonamides Trimethoprim	Altered bacterial target enzyme Altered bacterial target enzyme	Also resistant to cotrimoxazole
Other (see also Table 8.8)		
Chloroquine	Drug pumped out	Increasingly common

Antiviral therapy

There are far fewer antiviral than antibacterial drugs, because viruses have so few genes of their own and use mainly host mechanisms for their reproduction. Certain viral enzymes can be targeted, and the natural human product *interferon* (see Chapter 6) is now being produced commercially in huge amounts and has come into use in treating specific viruses, though its cost and unpleasant side-effects make it unsuitable for minor infections (Table 8.7).

Table 8.7 The antiviral drugs in current use

Drug	Site of action	Examples of clinical use
Amantadine	Blocks penetration	Influenza A
Acyclovir Vidarabine Gancyclovir Deoxycytidine	DNA polymerase DNA polymerase DNA polymerase	Herpes simplex, VZV Herpes simplex CMV Synergy with acyclovir, AZT
Zidovudine (AZT)	Reverse transcriptase	HIV
Interferon α	Viral RNA and protein synthesis; activation of CTL and NK cells	Hepatitis B, herpes

Therapy against protozoa, fungi, and worms

As might be expected, drugs that kill these eucaryotic organisms are also likely to damage their (eucaryotic) hosts (Table 8.8). Treatment of these infections usually needs to be prolonged, and is restricted by side-effects, sometimes very severe, as with the arsenic- and antimony-based drugs used against some protozoa. An exception is malaria, where the plant derivatives quinine, chloroquine, and artemisin are very effective, though resistance can develop. This is particularly serious in the case of chloroquine, the spread of resistance being helped by the fact that the malaria parasite has a well-developed sexual stage which allows new genes to travel rapidly through the population.

Table 8.8 Some drugs used for eucaryotic infections

Drug	Examples of clinical use
Antiprotozoal	
Primaquine	Liver-stage malaria
Quinine	Blood-stage malaria (acute)[1]
Chloroquine	Blood-stage malaria (prophylaxis)
Proguanil, mefloquine	Blood-stage malaria (prophylaxis)
Artemether	Blood-stage malaria (prophylaxis)
Metronidazole	Amoebiasis, giardiasis, trichomoniasis
Arsenicals	Trypanosomiasis
Antimonials	Leishmaniasis
Pentamidine	Toxoplasmosis, trypanosomiasis
Antifungal	
Griseofulvin	Dermatophytes
Amphotericin B	Cryptococcosis, coccidiomycosis, candidiasis
Trimethoprim	*Pneumocystis*
Pentamidine	*Pneumocystis*
Ketoconazole	Candidiasis, histoplasmosis, blastomycosis
Anthelminthic (anti-worm)	
Ivermectin	Nematodes, esp. filaria
Praziquantel	Schistosomiasis, tapeworms
Mebendazole	Nematodes

[1] *There is a large range of drugs against blood-stage malaria, to which parasites in different areas show different sensitivity patterns.*

INFECTION CONTROL: A COMPARISON OF METHODS

Every approach discussed in this chapter has its advantages and draw-backs, as summarized in Table 8.9. In an ideal world, public sanitation and awareness would be so high that infections would be rare. In the real world, vaccination has reduced the burden of infection, particularly with viruses, of which one has been eliminated and some half a dozen more may soon follow, but will probably never be as successful with bacteria and eucaryotes. Chemotherapy has had a dramatic effect on bacterial infection, but the emergence of resistant strains may justify the prediction of some pessimists that 'the golden age of antibiotics is over'. On the other hand, antibiotics are extremely profitable, which means that industry needs no encouragement to continue research into them, whereas vaccines are not, so that international support and encouragement, for example from agencies such as WHO, will always be required. Finally, it is worth mentioning that the public attitude to both vaccines and antibiotics is often very ill-informed, and health workers, as well as doctors, have a responsibility to know the facts and spell them out as calmly and accurately as possible.

Table 8.9 Control of infection: a comparison of available approaches

Method	Main usefulness
Personal precautions	Common respiratory and intestinal infections Sexually transmitted diseases
Safety routines	Hospital and laboratory infections
Public health measures	Food-, water-, and vector-borne diseases
Vaccination	Many viruses Some bacteria (esp. toxins)
Passive immunization	Post-exposure (esp. bacterial toxins) Hypogammaglobulinaemia
Chemotherapy	Most bacteria Some viruses Some protozoa, fungi, worms

FURTHER READING

Brown F, Dougan G, Hoey E M, Martin S J, Rima B K, Trudgett A 1993
Vaccine design. Wiley, Chichester, 130 pp
A look ahead at vaccines of the future.

HMSO 1988 Immunisation against infectious disease. HMSO, London, 117 pp
The 'little green book' on vaccines, used by the medical profession in the UK.

Inglis T J J, West A P 1995 Microbiology (colour guide). Churchill Livingstone,
Edinburgh, 137 pp

Lambert H P, O'Grady F W 1992 Antibiotic and chemotherapy, 6th edn.
Churchill Livingstone, Edinburgh, 561 pp
A massive review, medically oriented.

Maurer I M 1991 Hospital hygiene. Arnold, London, 152 pp

Moxon E R (ed) 1990 Modern vaccines. Arnold, London, 150 pp
A series of updated chapters from the Lancet.

Symonds J 1983 Notes on antimicrobial therapy. Churchill Livingstone,
Edinburgh, 105 pp
A shorter review of the subject.

Tutorial 8

Some questions on controlling infection that might turn up in either a microbiology or an immunology exam paper.

QUESTIONS

1. Distinguish between (1) disinfectants, (2) antiseptics, (3) antibiotics.

2. Why do you think there are no vaccines against (1) the common cold, (2) syphilis, (3) *Pneumocystis*?

3. In what conditions would measles vaccination be discouraged?

4. 'Penicillin has had its day.' Discuss.

5. Describe the uses and side-effects of (1) chloramphenicol, (2) isoniazid, (3) zidovudine (AZT), (4) quinine.

6. Smallpox has been eradicated. What other infectious diseases might follow?

ANSWERS

1. Disinfectants are used to kill organisms (mainly bacteria) on work surfaces, etc. They may be harmful to human tissues. Examples: phenol, hypochlorite. Antiseptics are also antibacterial, but safe to use on skin, wounds, etc. Examples: iodine, hydrogen peroxide. Antibiotics are chemotherapeutic drugs derived from living organisms. Examples: penicillin, streptomycin.

2. Colds are caused by a huge range of virus species and strains, each with different antigens which would need to be recognized by different lymphocytes, so it is hard to imagine a vaccine that would work against all of them. Syphilis is an example of a microorganism that appears to be resistant to all forms of immune attack. Also it is treatable by penicillin. The problem with *Pneumocystis* is that nothing is known about how normal individuals maintain immunity against it, and the vaccine would really only be needed for immunodeficient patients, who would probably not respond well.

3. The measles vaccine consists of living attenuated virus, so it should not be given to immunodeficient children, or to a patient undergoing immunosuppressive treatment. It is normally not given until about 15 months of age, because before that time residual maternally derived anti-measles antibody inhibits its action. A child known to be hypersensitive to egg proteins should be pretested with very small doses before being given the full vaccine.

4. There is plenty to discuss here. Strictly, the original drug penicillin G has indeed passed its peak. But modifications of it are very much in use today – benzylpenicillin, cloxacillin, ampicillin, to name but three. Bacteria resistant to all these (so-called methicillin-resistant because methicillin is used in the laboratory to test resistance) are an increasing problem in hospitals, but many bacteria have never developed resistance, for example *Neisseria* and most *Streptococci*.

5. Chloramphenicol is used against a wide range of bacteria, particularly in the eye and brain, but it suffers from the rare complication of bone marrow failure. Isoniazid is used in tuberculosis, usually with rifampicin and ethambutol. Treatment takes at least 6 months, and side-effects include skin rashes, neuropathy, and liver damage. Zidovudine is used in HIV infection, and patients have to be monitored for bone marrow failure (regular blood counts). Quinine was the first anti-malarial drug, but is nowadays reserved for acute life-threatening malaria. High doses can cause dizziness, deafness, blindness, and cardiac arrhythmias. Severe haemolytic anaemia ('blackwater fever') occasionally occurs following inadequate quinine treatment.

6. In the USA, it is predicted that polio, measles, mumps, and rubella may soon be eliminated, so the same is *possible* worldwide, though improbable in the short term. Diseases unlikely to be eliminated include those with many antigenic variants, those with a reservoir in animals, soil, water, etc., those which give rise to a carrier state, and those which the immune system cannot control at all, even when boosted. In practice, it is hard to imagine any infectious agent other than a virus being completely eradicated.

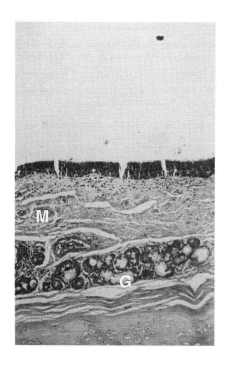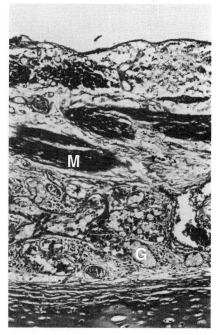

Microscope sections of the wall of a bronchus from a normal (left) and a chronic bronchitic lung (right, from a heavy smoker). The bronchitic section shows several changes, including hypertrophy of smooth muscle (M), hyperplasia of mucous glands (G), and squamous metaplasia of the surface epithelium. As described in this chapter, these changes are typical of the many possible adaptations to stress – in this case repeated irritation by cigarette smoke.

(Reproduced with kind permission from: Wheater P R, Burkitt H G, Stevens A, Lowe 1991 Basic histopathology: a colour atlas and text, 2nd edn. Churchill Livingstone, Edinburgh)

Adaptation to stress

9

■ CONTENTS

Case 9.1

A 70-year-old East African Asian man presented to his family practitioner with a 6-months' history of chronic cough. He had been a smoker for 40 years. He had contracted poliomyelitis in his childhood while living in Africa, which had resulted in wasting of his right leg. There was no other history. Chest X-ray did not reveal any specific abnormalities and bronchoscopy revealed changes in his bronchi which were reported by the pathologist as squamous metaplasia.

Most of us are aware of the changes that take place around us each day; the day turns to night and rain replaces brilliant sunshine. In the latter case, the first reaction is to reach for your umbrella and, failing that, to look for shelter. We are much less aware of the reactions that are continuously taking place within our own bodies owing to the changes occurring to our environment, both internally and externally. These adaptations may be subtle and only present at the metabolic level or may occur at the tissue or organ level, in which case they may be apparent to the naked eye. Here we will be concerned with changes at the cell and tissue level that take place as an adaptation to the changing conditions in which the cells find themselves.

Our East African patient had changes in his lungs called *metaplasia* which were an adaptation to his smoking, and he also had changes in his leg referred to as *atrophy*, which resulted from his polio infection. Both types of change are called *pathological adaptations*, since they result from an abnormal stress, induced accidentally or wilfully. There are also many adaptations that occur continuously because of normal changes within the body and these are called *physiological adaptations*. We will now consider these various types of adaptive response.

HYPERPLASIA AND HYPERTROPHY

Hyperplasia refers to an increase in the *number of cells* within tissues, while hypertrophy is an increase in the *cell size* (Fig. 9.1). In order to increase the cell number, cell division must take place, while the increased cell size in hypertrophy occurs without mitosis and cell replication. These adaptive responses are very common and occur in response to an increased functional demand on an organ or tissue. The type of demand that results in either hyperplasia or hypertrophy is essentially identical, and in many instances both occur together, the particular process being determined by the cell's ability to divide and replicate. Cardiac muscle, for instance, cannot replicate. Hence if increased demand is put on the heart in conditions like hypertension (raised blood pressure), the heart adapts by increasing the size of the cardiac muscle cells, and the ventricular wall becomes thicker – so-called left ventricular hypertrophy (LVH). As mentioned before, there are both physiological and pathological causes of these adaptive responses, so let us now consider some of these in more detail (Box 9.1).

Physiological hyperplasia and hypertrophy

Body-building

Anybody who has ever been involved in any kind of physical exercise will be familiar with this phenomenon. Tennis players, javelin throwers, and swimmers have hypertrophy of the shoulder girdle they depend so much on. An extreme example of skeletal hypertrophy is seen in professional body-builders, who selectively exercise various muscle groups in order to increase the bulk and definition of their muscles.

High-altitude training

Another example from training in athletes is the hyperplasia that occurs in the bone marrow of those living at high altitudes. Decreased oxygen in the

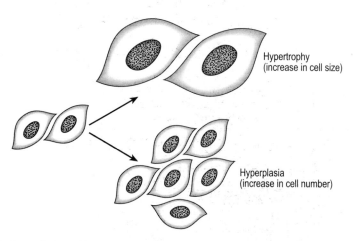

Fig. 9.1 Hyperplasia and hypertrophy.

■ **BOX 9.1 Hyperplasia and hypertrophy**

Some examples:

Bone marrow hyperplasia
Hormonal
    Breast enlargement at puberty and pregnancy
    Uterine enlargement at pregnancy
    Endometrial hyperplasia
    Adrenal hyperplasia
    Thyroid hyperplasia
Liver hyperplasia following injury
Myocardial hypertrophy
Muscular hypertrophy in athletes
Prostatic hyperplasia and hypertrophy
Proliferative vascular disease, e.g. retina in diabetes
Wound healing with hyperplasia of epidermis and connective tissue

air at altitude leads to production of the hormone erythropoietin in the kidney, which brings about an increase in red blood cell production from the marrow. This physiological adaptation is exploited by athletes, and is the reason why many train at high altitude prior to competition: it boosts their red blood cell numbers and hence their oxygen-carrying capacity which is so vital for competitive exertion.

Puberty and pregnancy

The breast is really a modified sweat gland which undergoes tremendous changes during puberty and pregnancy. Under the influence of hormones such as oestrogens and progestagens, the breast tissue undergoes hyperplasia at puberty to form the adult female breast. The cyclical changes in the hormone levels are also influential during the menstrual cycle, and the breast tissue undergoes additional proliferation during this period. The other main episode in the life of the breast comes at the time of pregnancy, when the breast prepares for lactation. This hyperplasia and hypertrophy are also under the influence of hormones such as prolactin and growth hormone.

During pregnancy, the uterus changes from a pear-sized organ to one that can carry and deliver a baby of 2–3 kg. This change occurs by an increase in both size and number of the smooth muscle cells within the myometrium. This organ is fascinating because, when the baby has been delivered, the uterus will shrink back down again, so you would never guess that it had been pregnant. This reversibility is one of the hallmarks of adaptive responses. The changes only last as long as the stimulus is present and disappear when the stimulus is removed. This differentiates them from neoplastic proliferations, which we will consider in Chapter 12.

A Greek myth – or was it?

There is a very interesting example of hyperplasia that was well known to even the ancient Greeks. The story of Prometheus states that when he upset the god Zeus, he was tied up to a stake on the mountain and each day a vulture came and tore at his liver. The pain went on day after day, because each night the liver grew back! Maybe the story is a myth, but there is nothing mythical about the ability of the liver to regenerate. It does exactly that, by division of the surviving cells. What is amazing is that it knows when to stop. If you chop off a bit of the liver at operation, it will in time grow back to the right size, so that you would never know the operation had been carried out at all. Unfortunately the same does not apply to all organs: for example, heart and kidney cells do not regenerate.

Pathological hyperplasia and hypertrophy

Although it is customary to divide these responses into physiological and pathological, the distinction may not always be clear-cut. When does a physiological response of the myocardium to raised blood pressure become pathological? A useful definition is that if the changes allow the tissue to work or cope better, they are physiological; when they no longer fulfil a purpose, they become pathological. Let us consider some more obvious examples of pathological responses.

Prostatic enlargement

Like the breast, the prostate is also an 'endocrine organ' and sensitive to changes in the hormones within the body. Practically all men are destined to dribble through old age as hormonal changes lead to hyperplasia and hypertrophy of the gland. The differing responses of the tissues within the gland lead to nodular proliferations which may impinge on the urethra and create a 'ball valve' effect and hence interrupt micturition. Though they are due to a physiological change in hormones, there is no obvious benefit from either the hormonal changes or the response of the prostate.

Myocardial infarction

When the blood supply to the myocardial cells is interrupted by coronary artery disease or thrombosis, the myocardial cells die unless the supply is reinstated quickly. The myocardial cells do not have a capacity to regenerate and instead they are replaced by scar tissue, which consists of hyperplasia within the connective tissue elements, as fibroblasts and myofibroblasts increase in number to replace the dead myocardial cells. If the damage is substantial, the remaining myocardium may not be able to cope with the workload, in which case it will try to compensate by hyper-trophy of the remaining myocardial cells. Of course this cannot go on indefinitely, which is why eventually the myocardium fails. Bypass grafts are simply a way of replumbing the system so that the remaining myocardium receives enough blood to stay alive and carry out its normal function (see also Chapter 11).

Cushing's syndrome

This syndrome is due to excessive glucocorticoid secretion and results in central obesity, hirsutism (excess hair), high blood pressure, diabetes and osteoporosis. One of the main causes is an ACTH (adrenocorticotrophic hormone) secreting tumour of the pituitary. The excess ACTH over-stimulates the cortex of the adrenal gland, which undergoes hyperplasia, leading to secretion of excess glucocorticoid hormones. Removal of the pituitary tumour will allow the adrenal gland to revert back to normal.

ATROPHY

Physiological atrophy

Atrophy is a decrease in the size of a tissue and is brought about by a decrease in *cell size* and/or *numbers* (Fig. 9.2). The mechanism is very often apoptosis (pronounced *apo*-tosis; the other name is programmed cell death, as described in Chapter 2). This type of adaptation occurs because of a decrease in the body's requirement for certain functions. Just as an enlargement in tissues can occur by both increased growth and decreased death, so the decrease in tissue size occurs by increased death as well as decreased growth. In both cases it is the balance between the two processes that matters.

Physiological atrophy occurs during embryogenesis (e.g. the disappearance of branchial cleft and thyroglossal duct), during the neonatal period (atrophy of umbilical cord after birth), and also during old age. The term *hypoplasia* is often used synonymously with atrophy, although strictly speaking it means a failure to grow to a normal size, and therefore refers mainly to problems during embryogenesis and the neonatal period. Let us consider some examples of atrophy (Box 9.2).

The thymus

The thymus gland is a good example of a tissue that undergoes physiological atrophy. It is a lymphoid organ that is crucial for the development and processing of T lymphocytes (see Chapter 5). The activity of the organ is maximal in the fetus and early childhood and the gland undergoes atrophy quite rapidly after puberty, though it never disappears completely.

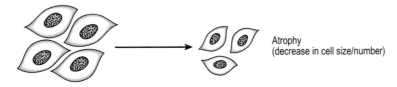

Atrophy
(decrease in cell size/number)

Fig. 9.2 Atrophy.

■ **BOX 9.2 Causes of atrophy**

Embryological development and morphogenesis
  Branchial cleft
  Ductus arteriosus
  Thymus

Decreased demand and workload
  Physical
  Hormonal
  Ageing
  Immobilization as in fracture healing

Loss of blood supply
  Peripheral vascular disease

Loss of innervation
  Polio
  Neurodegenerative disorder

Poor nutrition

The genital system

Following the menopause and the decrease in female hormones, there is no longer a requirement for the endometrium and uterus to wait in readiness for an expected pregnancy. They therefore undergo atrophy by a decrease in cell size and number. Similarly, the testes in males undergo atrophy with age, although the exact timing of the 'male menopause' is more difficult to define.

Bone

One of the distressing effects of the menopause and the associated loss of oestrogens is the profound loss of bone density that occurs in women. This loss of bone density – called *osteoporosis* – has a significant effect and is responsible for the loss of height (as vertebra get smaller) and fractures seen with advancing age. Osteoporosis occurs in both sexes, but the effects are more dramatic in women. Hormone replacement therapy (HRT) has been shown to reverse this effect on bone loss. This type of treatment is still not used widely owing to the suspect role of HRT in malignant transformation, particularly in the uterus. The risks, however, are small if it is not used continuously for more than 5–10 years. When HRT is stopped, bone loss will recur.

Pathological atrophy

This usually occurs because of loss of function of a part of the body for reasons such as damage to the blood supply or loss of nerve innervation (Box 9.2).

Fracture

Most people will be familiar with the effects of having a limb in plaster following a fracture (the healing of fractures is discussed in Chapter 2). When the plaster is removed, the most dramatic effect is the loss of muscle bulk from the limb, and in an athlete the difference between the two sides can be striking. The disuse of the muscle due to the plaster cast leads to atrophy of the muscles. With physiotherapy and hard work, the muscle bulk will of course return. As with hypertrophy and hyperplasia, removing the stimulus for the process does reverse the situation.

Loss of nerve and blood supply

Our patient from East Africa had a wasted leg due to poliomyelitis in his youth. This is an example of atrophy due to loss of nerve innervation. Polio causes damage to the peripheral nerves; hence the muscles normally innervated by those nerves undergo atrophy in the absence of stimulation. Loss of blood supply has a similar effect since the tissues and organs can no longer get the nutrition they need to maintain cellular metabolism. Both these factors may also be important in the type of atrophy referred to as 'pressure atrophy'. A tumour, for instance, may obstruct the blood supply or destroy nerve innervation to a particular tissue, causing atrophy of that part. Another common example is the *bedsore* that occurs in immobile patients, particularly if there is wasting of the tissues, as in the elderly or debilitated. This is why it is so important for the position of the bedridden patient to be changed frequently.

Endocrine-related atrophy

You will remember that we discussed Cushing's syndrome, where there was hyperplasia due to overproduction of ACTH. The opposite effect is a decreased production of ACTH due to destruction of the pituitary gland either by tumour or vascular accident. This results in decreased stimulation of the adrenal gland and hence atrophy. Excess exogenous administration of steroid hormones will have a similar effect, by blocking the production of ACTH from the pituitary. Note that in Addison's disease the destruction of the adrenal cortex and decreased secretion of cortisol is due to auto-immunity (Chapter 7).

METAPLASIA

This is defined as the transformation of one type of normal differentiated cell into another differentiated cell type (Fig. 9.3). Like the processes discussed earlier, it is a reversible adaptive response to stress induced in a particular tissue (Box 9.3). The new cell type is designed to be better able to cope with the environmental stress which led to the response.

Smoking and squamous metaplasia

Our East African patient also had squamous metaplasia of the bronchial mucosa, related to smoking. When long-term smokers present with chronic

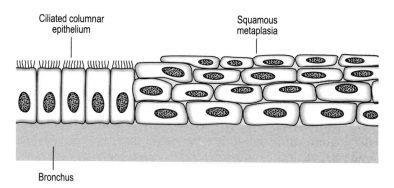

Fig. 9.3 Metaplasia.

■ **BOX 9.3 Examples of metaplasia**

Squamous metaplasia
   Cervix
   Bronchus
   Prostate
   Kidneys
   Bladder
   Breast

Glandular metaplasia
   Gastric type in oesophagus
   Intestinal type in stomach

Osseous and chondroid metaplasia
   Soft tissue
   Bladder
   Kidney
   Breast

Others
   Apocrine metaplasia in breast
   Metaplastic tissues in tumours

cough, the first worry is whether they have a carcinoma. In this case, only metaplasia was found on biopsy. The irritant effect of smoke on the respiratory ciliated epithelium converts it to a more hardy squamous epithelium which is not normally found at this site. Metaplasia is a benign condition and there are no sinister implications from the diagnosis of metaplastic epithelium. However, it does allow an occurrence of a tumour type that normally does not exist at that location, since once squamous epithelium has developed at this site by metaplasia, it is possible for squamous cell carcinoma to occur in the lung. The process of metaplasia itself is not precancerous but, once the epithelium is there, it is available for the genetic mutations that lead a cell from normal to cancerous (Chapter 12).

Other examples of squamous metaplasia

Squamous metaplasia can also occur in the bladder, where, owing to chronic inflammation of infection with schistosomiasis (a tropical worm infection), the transitional epithelium undergoes transformation. The ducts in the pancreas and the bile ducts can also undergo similar changes as a result of chronic inflammation set up by the presence of gallstones.

Glandular metaplasia

Although squamous metaplasia is the commonest type of transformation observed, there are other types that occur in special circumstances. During reflux of acid from the stomach into the oesophagus ('heartburn'), damage to the oesophageal squamous epithelium leads to a glandular metaplasia. The columnar glandular epithelium of the stomach is much more resistant to acid owing to its ability to secrete mucus, and hence reflux leads to a gastric type of glandular metaplasia in the oesophagus. This condition is known as Barrett's oesophagus. Hence, while squamous carcinomas are the major variant in the oesophagus, in Barrett's oesophagus the patient may get adenocarcinomas (see Chapter 12 for details of the classification of tumours).

Mesenchymal metaplasia

Metaplastic changes can also be identified in connective tissue. For example, bony (osseous) metaplasia can be seen in degenerate tissues such as atheroma and necrotic foci. This type of change is also observed in some tumours, but by definition the term metaplasia refers to mature tissues and not to malignant tissues. The calcification that may also occur is not due to metaplasia, and is discussed in Chapter 10.

In summary, the body adapts to various stresses within its internal environment by changes in the cells and tissues that allow it to cope better with the insult. If the stress is withdrawn, the tissues go back to their original state. The body's ability to cope with these stresses is not infinite, and if they escalate beyond the ability to cope, the tissues or organs will fail in their function, as occurs with cardiac failure following long-term untreated hypertension. The important thing to remember is that the body is constantly adapting to a constantly changing environment.

Tutorial 9

Test your grasp of adaptive responses by answering the following questions. Remember that you may not find all the answers in this chapter, and a bit of cross-reading may be needed.

QUESTIONS

1. What are hyperplasia and hypertrophy? Can you think of two conditions in which there is pure hyperplasia or hypertrophy, and two in which they occur together?

2. What is atrophy? Give some examples. How does it differ from involution?

3. Define metaplasia. What type of metaplasia would you expect in the cervix following inflammation? Name some other types of metaplasia with examples. How does it differ from dysplasia?

4. How does hyperplasia differ from a benign neoplasm?

ANSWERS

1. Hyperplasia is an increase in cell number and hypertrophy is an increase in cell size. Examples of pure hyperplasia include hyperplasia of bone marrow cells at high altitude and hyperplasia of breast epithelium at puberty. By contrast, the increased muscle bulk following exercise is an example of pure hypertrophy. Mixed hyperplasia and hypertrophy is commoner and examples include prostatic enlargement and uterine enlargement in pregnancy.

2. Atrophy is a decrease in the size of organs or tissues as a result of a decrease in cell size and number. Examples include loss of muscle bulk after fracture and plaster cast, loss of innervation or blood supply to tissues and organs that can occur with diseases such as poliomyelitis, and peripheral vascular disease. Involution is essentially another name for atrophy. In certain circumstances, such as the thymus shrinking with age or the uterus after birth, the term involution is more often used, but the underlying process is the same.

3. Metaplasia is a change from one type of normal epithelium to another normal type. The cervix undergoes squamous metaplasia. The glandular epithelium of the endocervix will transform to the squamous epithelium which is normally found at the ectocervix. Other examples of metaplasia include squamous metaplasia in the bronchus, gastric metaplasia in oesophagus and osseous metaplasia in soft tissues. In the breast, the ductal epithelium may exhibit apocrine metaplasia, where the cells become large

and pink with abundant cytoplasm. The aetiology is unclear. Almost all organs in the body exhibit one or other type of metaplastic change. Try listing these for the different body systems!

Dysplasia is a difficult term and refers to atypical cytological and morphological characteristics of cells and tissues, which gives it a neoplastic connotation. It is therefore premalignant. However, mild degrees of dysplasia may be reversible. See Chapter 12 for more details.

4. Hyperplasia is an increase in cell number, which also occurs in neoplastic proliferation. However, hyperplasia is a reaction to a stimulus and is an adaptive phenomenon, and will regress when the stimulus is removed. A neoplasm, on the other hand, is by definition autonomous and even when the stimulus that started it off is removed, it continues to grow. A neoplasm is also clonal (that is, derived from a single parent cell) and all the cells in the lesion show an identical genetic pattern; hyperplasia, however, is polyclonal and composed of a mixture of cells from different parent cells. (See Chapter 12 for more details of dysplasia, neoplasia, and other matters concerning tumours.)

FURTHER READING

Cotran R S, Kumar V, Robbins S L 1994 Pathological basis of disease, 5th edn. Saunders, Philadelphia

Lakhani S R, Dilly S A, Finlayson C J 1993 Basic pathology: an introduction to the mechanisms of disease. Arnold, London

Stevens A, Lowe J 1995 Pathology. Mosby, London

Underwood J C E 1996 General and systemic pathology, 2nd edn. Churchill Livingstone, Edinburgh

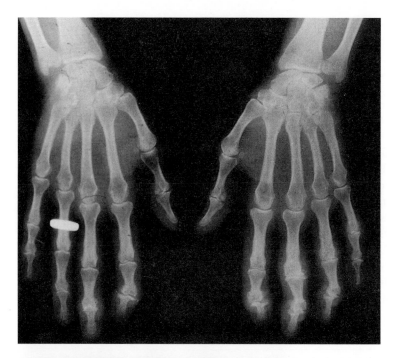

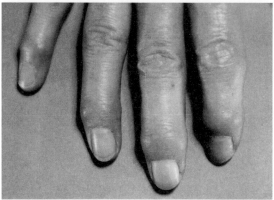

Compare these hands with those shown at the beginning of Chapter 7. Note that here the damage is mainly to the terminal finger joints. This is osteoarthritis, and the pathology is quite different from that in rheumatoid arthritis, being simply the result of repeated use – in other words a degenerative disease. In this chapter we consider some common degenerative diseases, and also some other conditions in which damage is to normal metabolic processes rather than to whole tissues.

(Reproduced with kind permission of Dr Michael Shipley, Dept of Rheumatology, UCL Hospital NHS Trust, London.)

Metabolic and degenerative diseases

■ CONTENTS

Case 10.1

A 62-year-old hypertensive man presented to his general practitioner with a painful toe. On examination, his right big toe was swollen, red, and extremely tender to touch. He had been hypertensive for over 10 years and had been taking thiazide diuretics to control his blood pressure. The doctor diagnosed gout and this was confirmed on aspiration of the joint and microscopy.

Almost every disease has some effect on metabolic processes and leads to some damage of tissues. But in certain diseases a metabolic abnormality is the dominant effect, and in others we see more or less pure tissue damage. These disorders therefore constitute a heterogeneous group, and it is clearly impossible to discuss them all. In this chapter, we will consider two of the important acquired metabolic disorders, namely diabetes and gout. We will also look at one of the commonest forms of degenerative arthropathy – osteoarthritis – and then discuss disorders related to deposition of amyloid, calcium, and iron in tissues.

DIABETES

The characteristic feature of this disease is an insufficiency of insulin, which leads to hyperglycaemia (raised blood glucose) and glycosuria (glucose in urine). The disorder can be *primary* or *secondary*. Primary diabetes is much commoner and diabetes secondary to other diseases is rare. Primary diabetes is further subdivided into insulin-dependent diabetes mellitus (*IDDM or type 1*) and non-insulin-dependent diabetes mellitus (*NIDDM or type 2*).

Diabetes occurring in young people below the age of 20 years (juvenile-onset) is almost always type 1 (IDDM), while that occurring in older people is generally of type 2 (NIDDM). Type 1 IDDM has an inherited predisposition associated with HLA-DR3 and DR4 (see Chapter 7 for the significance of this). There is also some evidence to suggest that a viral infection is responsible for initiating the destruction of the β-cells via an autoimmune mechanism. Antibodies to Coxsackie B and mumps virus have been detected in patients with IDDM. Type 2 NIDDM is not associated with a genetic predisposition and there is a resistance to insulin at the tissue level rather than a lack of the hormone.

The damage to tissues in diabetes is believed to occur via the binding of glucose to tissue proteins (glycosylation). This inhibits the normal function of the proteins. Some tissues, such as the lens in the eye and neurones, are able to metabolize the glucose into sorbitol and fructose, which accumulates and causes swelling (oedema) of the tissues and even cell death. As we have seen in previous chapters, damage to cells and tissues leads to the process of inflammation and subsequent healing and repair, some of which may take the form of scarring and fibrosis.

Complications of diabetes

With this background, it is easy to appreciate the diverse range of manifestations observed in patients with long-standing IDDM. These complications include an increased propensity for atheroma (see Chapter 11) and hence ischaemic heart disease, renal glomerular damage and kidney failure, eye damage due to haemorrhage and by proliferation of new vessels in the retina, cataract formation, an increased susceptibility to infection and diabetic coma. These complications are summarized in Figure 10.1. About 15% of patients needing a kidney graft (Chapter 7) have diabetic renal failure.

GOUT

Gout results from high levels of uric acid in the blood. Most of the uric acid is derived as a breakdown product of purines. Purines are derived from nucleic acids (from DNA, RNA) when cells are broken down. A small amount of uric acid is derived from dietary sources (e.g. meat). The uric acid in the blood is transported to the kidney where it is excreted. A schematic pathway of uric acid metabolism is illustrated in Figure 10.2.

Gout may either be *primary*, due to a genetic abnormality of the purine metabolism pathway, or *secondary*, due to excess production of uric acid. An example of primary gout is the Lesch-Nyhan syndrome. In this disorder, children develop gout owing to a deficiency of hypoxanthine guanine phosphoribosyl transferase (HGPRT – Fig. 10.2). Secondary gout may arise when there is excessive tissue destruction. A good example of this is tissue breakdown following chemotherapy for cancer. Here, a large number of cells will be lysed in a relatively short time, producing huge amounts of uric acid. If there is renal insufficiency (this may also be a side-effect of chemotherapy drugs), gout becomes a significant complication.

Gout is much more common in men than women. Other risk factors include a positive family history, a large body size, and a diet with excessive alcohol and red meat.

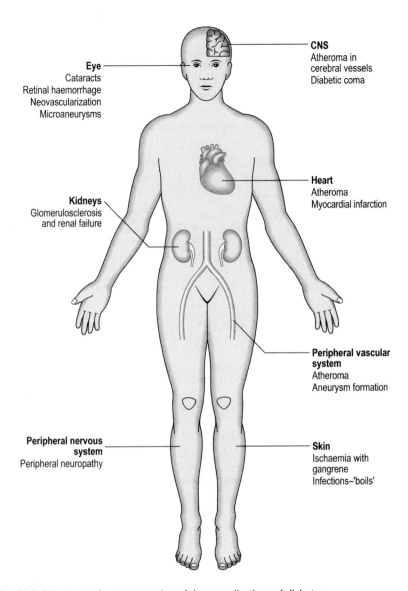

Fig. 10.1 Diagrammatic representation of the complications of diabetes.

Complications of gout

The main complications (and hence clinical manifestations) of gout are due to excess uric acid in the blood. It is present as monosodium urate within the blood, and excess levels lead to deposition of these urate crystals in various tissues. Deposits in soft tissues are called tophi and may be characteristically found in ear lobes as well as other sites. Deposits in joints set off an inflammatory response which results in painful synovitis and arthritis (as in the example at the beginning of the chapter). Deposition may also occur in the kidney, leading to urate stones and kidney damage, which further aggravate the condition.

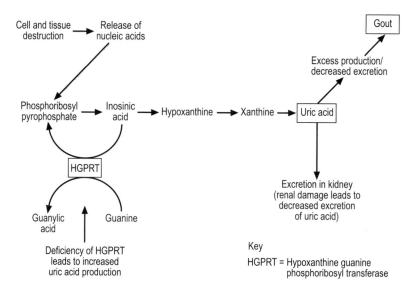

Fig. 10.2 Uric acid metabolism. Destruction of cells releases nucleic acids which are metabolized to uric acid. Increased production, decreased excretion, or lack of HGPRT leads to increased accumulation of uric acid and hence gout.

OSTEOARTHRITIS

Osteoarthritis (OA) is an extremely common degenerative disease that causes considerable morbidity. It generally affects the large weight-bearing joints (from 'wear and tear'), although other joints may be involved, particularly after suffering trauma. The most important symptoms resulting from OA are pain, reduced movement and deformity of the affected joint.

For many patients, there are no specific predisposing factors. In some specialized circumstance, a predisposing factor is obvious. Athletes who sustain injury to their joints – e.g. repeated knee or ankle injury – are likely to develop OA in those joints. Previous chronic inflammatory arthritis due to gout or rheumatoid arthritis for example, will also predispose to the development of secondary OA.

The pathological change in OA resides in the articular cartilage. Initially the cartilage becomes irregular and fibrillary. Eventually there is loss of the cartilage and, in severe cases, the full thickness of the cartilage may be lost. This leads in turn to changes in the bone underneath the cartilage. The bone proliferates as a response to the damage and this leads to increased distortion of the shape of the joint, further accelerating the damage to the articular cartilage. Excessive bony proliferation produces spurs of bone called *osteophytes*, which are the hallmark of OA. It is these osteophytes that are responsible for the limitation of movement that eventually occurs. When present as nodules around the distal joints of the fingers, they are called 'Heberden's nodes'.

Complications of OA

There are no systemic complications of OA. The main problems are related to pain, deformity, and lack of the range of movement in the affected joint. As OA becomes severe, it leads to immobility, especially when the affected joints are the hip, knee, and ankle. Although the synovium is not generally inflamed, there may be an effusion within the joint which also contributes to the reduction in movement of the joint. Note that the disease rheumatoid arthritis (see Chapter 7) is different in many respects, and does have serious systemic consequences.

TISSUE DEPOSITION DISEASES

Amyloidosis

Amyloid is an extracellular deposit of proteinaceous material. Rudolf Virchow coined and popularized the term 'amyloid' because of the reaction of the material with iodine and sulphuric acid, an indication that the material is 'starch-like'. The amyloid itself is not toxic but it causes damage by producing atrophy of cells and tissues through pressure or ischaemia, or by interfering with function of the tissues.

Amyloid deposition may be *localized* or *systemic*. Although all types of amyloid look the same microscopically, there are in fact many different types with a different composition. All of them, however, share the properties of having a β-pleated sheet structure, a fibrillary ultrastructure, and extracellular deposition. For unknown reasons, the β-pleated structure prevents the material from being digested and removed by phagocytic cells. There are two protein components in amyloid, the variable component and a glycoprotein common to all amyloid except cerebral amyloid, which is called *amyloid P-component*.

Table 10.1 shows a simplified classification of amyloidosis. Only amyloid related to immune disorders (AL) and amyloid related to chronic reactive conditions (AA) are reasonably common and cause significant disease.

Systemic amyloidosis

AL: immune-associated amyloid. Although the reactive type (AA – see below) of amyloid is most common worldwide, the AL form is commonest in developed countries. This type of amyloid is associated with plasma cell disorders, e.g. multiple myeloma. Approximately 6–15% of patients with myeloma develop amyloid and most will die within a year of diagnosis, 50% of them from heart failure. AL amyloid is so designated because it is derived from the *light* chains of immunoglobulin molecules.

AA: reactive amyloid. This type of amyloid is called secondary or reactive amyloid because it is associated with chronic infective or inflammatory disorders, such as rheumatoid arthritis, tuberculosis, chronic inflammatory bowel disease, and osteomyelitis. Approximately 10% of patients with rheumatoid arthritis will develop amyloid, generally after 10–15 years of

Table 10.1 Classification of amyloid

	Type	Protein
Systemic		
Immune disorders, e.g. myeloma	AL	Immunoglobulin light chains
Reactive	AA	Serum amyloid A associated protein
Familial		
Neuropathic	AF	Transthyretin
Non-neuropathic	AA	Serum amyloid A associated protein
Haemodialysis-associated	AH	β2 microglobulin
Senile	ASc	Transthyretin
Localized		
Cerebral		
Alzheimer's disease		
Down's syndrome	A4 β-protein	–
Endocrine-related	AE	Calcitonin, insulin, etc.
Cutaneous	AD	?Keratin
Plasmacytoma	AL	Immunoglobulin light chains

active rheumatoid disease. The kidney is most commonly affected (70%), and half of the patients will die from the effects of amyloid within 5 years.

Amyloid A protein is not derived from immunoglobulins but from a protein which is produced by the liver and is one of the acute phase proteins.

AF: familial amyloid. The amyloid in this disorder is deposited principally in nerves (familial amyloid polyneuropathy). It has an autosomal dominant pattern of inheritance. The genetic abnormality affects the production of transthyretin (prealbumin), whose normal role is the *trans*port of *thy*roxin and *retin*ol; hence the name. The abnormal transthyretin molecules can aggregate to form amyloid fibrils.

AH: haemodialysis-associated amyloid. Patients receiving *haemodialysis* for chronic renal failure may get this type of amyloidosis, which particularly affects the joints and tendons and may cause carpal tunnel syndrome. There is an accumulation of β2 microglobulin because this molecule is not filtered during haemodialysis (β2 microglobulin is a normal serum protein).

ASc: senile amyloid. This form of amyloid deposition is generally asymptomatic except for occasional cases of senile cardiac amyloid. The amyloid protein is formed from an abnormal transthyretin molecule, indicating a genetic predisposition.

Localized amyloidosis

Cerebral amyloid. Cerebral amyloid differs from other forms of amyloid in that it does not contain component P and it can occur in intracellular (neurofibrillary tangles) as well as extracellular locations. The significance of cerebral amyloid is unclear, but it occurs in Alzheimer's dementia, Down's syndrome, and some elderly normal individuals. The amyloid may be deposited in vessel walls and neurofibrillary tangles.

AE: endocrine-related amyloid. Certain endocrine tumours, such as islet cell tumours of the pancreas, contain amyloid derived from the hormone or prohormone produced at that site. Thus, in islet cell tumours, insulin and proinsulin are implicated. The amyloid does not appear to have any clinical significance.

Other types of amyloidosis are rare and of uncertain significance.

Demonstration of amyloid in tissues

At autopsy, amyloid can be demonstrated in fresh organ slices by applying 1% acetic acid followed by iodine. Amyloid, if present will stain a deep brown colour, which will turn blue-violet when 10% sulphuric acid is added. In formalin-fixed, paraffin-embedded tissue sections, amyloid may be demonstrated using Congo red. When viewed under polarized light amyloid gives an apple-green colour. Alternatively, specific antisera to the different forms of amyloid may be used on tissue sections by the immuno-peroxidase technique.

Calcification

Tissue calcification can be divided into (1) dystrophic calcification and (2) metastatic calcification

Table 10.2 summarizes the features of the two types of calcification. Dystrophic calcification occurs in tissues that are dying or are non-viable following some type of injury, involution, or alteration. The serum calcium is normal, which contrasts with metastatic calcification, where the serum calcium levels are high and calcification occurs in normal tissues.

Table 10.2 Types of calcification

Dystrophic	Metastatic
Tissues affected are damaged or dead	Tissues affected are normal prior to calcification
Serum calcium level is normal	Serum calcium is elevated
Examples of tissues affected include scars, tumours, atheroma, damaged heart valves, necrotic nodes (e.g. after tuberculosis). Almost every organ may therefore be involved	Examples of tissues affected include kidneys, soft tissues, blood vessels
	Causes of raised calcium include: Primary and tertiary hyperparathyroidism Bony metastasis, myeloma, sarcoidosis Chronic renal failure

Dystrophic calcification can be intra- or extracellular and may progress to bone formation (osseous metaplasia: Chapter 9). The mechanism of dystrophic calcification involves two stages: initiation followed by propagation. When cells or tissues die or undergo necrosis, large amounts of calcium enter the cell as the membrane ionic pumps fail. This calcium combines with phosphates within the mitochondria to produce the hydroxyapatite crystals. After this initiation, the propagation of crystal formation depends on the local concentration of calcium and phosphate. Generally dystrophic calcification acts only as a sign of previous injury but at certain sites, such as the heart valves, it may also interfere with function.

In contrast, metastatic calcification results from an abnormality of calcium metabolism with high levels of serum calcium. Causes of hypercalcaemia include primary and tertiary hyperparathyroidism, hyperthyroidism, sarcoidosis, cancer metastasizing to bone, and excess vitamin D ingestion. This form of calcification can occur in normal tissues. Common sites include soft tissues, blood vessels, lungs, and kidneys. The actual mechanism of the calcification is similar to the dystrophic variety.

Iron deposition

When excess iron accumulates in the body, it is deposited within the macrophages of the reticuloendothelial system (lymph nodes, bone marrow, spleen, and Kupffer cells of the liver). It also accumulates within the parenchymal cells of various organs, most notably the pancreas, liver, and heart. Deposition of iron in the pancreas leads to destruction of islet cells, resulting in diabetes. Iron deposition in the liver may also have serious consequences, since it is toxic to liver cells and leads to cell death with subsequent scarring and fibrosis. If left untreated, cirrhosis will ensue. A complication of cirrhosis is carcinoma of the liver (hepatocellular carcinoma). Heart failure may also occur in severe cases owing to deposition of iron in myocardial cells, necrosis, and, ultimately, fibrosis.

Excess iron deposition, termed *haemochromatosis*, can be divided into *primary* and *secondary*. Primary haemochromatosis is inherited as an autosomal recessive disorder and has an association with HLA-A3, B7, and B14. Males are affected more than females (7:1). Complications of primary haemochromatosis are summarized in Figure 10.3. Secondary haemochromatosis may occur as a result of haemolytic anaemias, liver disease, or high iron ingestion. The other form of systemic iron overload is much less severe and is termed *haemosiderosis*. It results from similar causes to secondary haemochromatosis, but the excess iron is not sufficient to overburden the macrophages and deposition in parenchymal cells does not occur. It results from an imbalance between the amount of iron ingested and the amount excreted.

Iron is an important element in the body with well-known roles in haemoglobin and myoglobin synthesis. Many enzymes also need iron for proper function. Approximately 80% of the body's iron is in one of these functional forms while the remaining 20% is stored as ferritin or haemosiderin. There is no control over the excretion of iron and so the total iron in the body is regulated by its absorption. Some iron is lost through loss of cells at epithelial surfaces and small amounts of blood are lost in the gastrointestinal tract. Menstruation is an important source of iron loss in

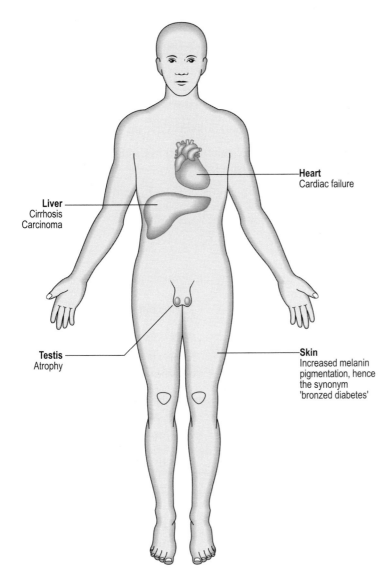

Heart
Cardiac failure

Liver
Cirrhosis
Carcinoma

Testis
Atrophy

Skin
Increased melanin
pigmentation, hence
the synonym
'bronzed diabetes'

Fig. 10.3 Diagrammatic representation of the complications of haemochromatosis. The clinical effects are due to excess deposition of iron in tissues.

premenopausal women and may account for the higher incidence of haemochromatosis in men.

Once the iron has been absorbed in excess, as in primary haemochromatosis, it accumulates in the parenchymal cells of various organs. It appears that the iron may have a role in the production of free radicals which damage the cell membranes and organelles. Iron also tends to accumulate in the lysosomes, and any damage to the lysosomal membrane will release degradative enzymes which could also damage cellular components and lead to cell death. However, cell death is not inevitable and the risks can be reduced with iron-chelating drugs such as desferrioxamine, which binds iron and is then excreted in the urine.

Tutorial 10

QUESTIONS

1. Draw up a table comparing osteoarthritis and rheumatoid arthritis.

2. What are inborn errors of metabolism? Give an example.

3. List some of the common pigments seen in tissue sections and describe how they may be distinguished.

4. What do you understand by 'fatty change'? List the causes of fatty change.

ANSWERS

1. The most important distinguishing features are as follows:

Osteoarthritis	*Rheumatoid arthritis*
Involves articular cartilage	Involves synovial membrane
Main abnormality is *degeneration* of cartilage	Main abnormality is *inflammation* of synovial membrane
Affects any age but mainly middle to elderly	Affects any age
Mainly large weight-bearing joints	Usually small joints of hand and feet
Often single joint involvement	Usually multiple joints
Pre-existing trauma or occupation history important	No previous history of trauma, etc.
No systemic symptoms	A systemic disease with raised ESR, anaemia, positive rheumatoid factors, and other associated disorders – e.g. pericarditis, lung disease

2. Inborn errors of metabolism are inherited disorders due to a single gene defect. They manifest in infancy or childhood and are a rare but important cause of illness. They result from defects in enzymes that are required for protein synthesis.

Examples include phenylketonuria, homocystinuria, and the porphyrias. For example, in phenylketonuria, which is autosomal recessive, there is a deficiency of phenylalanine hydroxylase. This enzyme converts phenylalanine to tyrosine. If untreated, the child will develop hair and skin depigmentation, cerebral fits, and mental retardation. Treatment consists of a diet low in phenylalanine. In the UK, screening is carried out on all infants with the Guthrie test.

3. We have already considered some of these, e.g. iron and calcium. Iron appears brown in tissue sections, as does lipofuscin and melanin. Iron is demonstrated by Prussian blue stain, which makes it appear blue in sections. It is important to distinguish melanin from iron since it is seen in naevi and in malignant melanoma. It can be stained black with the Masson-Fontana stain. Lipofuscin, which is a 'wear and tear' pigment due to oxidation of lipids, can be stained black by Sudan black stain. Calcification is usually obvious in sections as it has a crystalline and laminated appearance, but it can be stained with von Kossa's stain when it appears black. Bile pigment also appears brown or green-yellow in ordinary haematoxylin and eosin (H&E) stained sections. Fouchet technique stains the bile green.

4. Fatty change refers to an excess of intracellular lipid (fat) within the cytoplasm. This gives the cell a bubbly appearance. It is a non-specific reaction to a variety of insults, and is completely reversible. Sometimes it is present adjacent to tissues that are more severely damaged or show frank evidence of necrosis. Fatty change can occur in any organ but is most frequent in the liver, as the liver is the major site of lipid metabolism. Causes include alcohol ingestion, protein malnutrition, diabetes, pregnancy, ischaemia, obesity, and drugs such as steroids.

FURTHER READING

Lacy P 1995 Treating diabetes with transplanted cells. Scientific American July, pp 40–46

Shipley M 1993 A colour atlas of rheumatology, 3rd edn. Wolfe, London, 175 pp

Underwood J C E 1996 General and systemic pathology, 2nd edn. Churchill Livingstone, Edinburgh, 941 pp

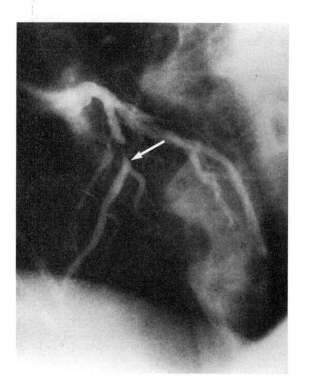
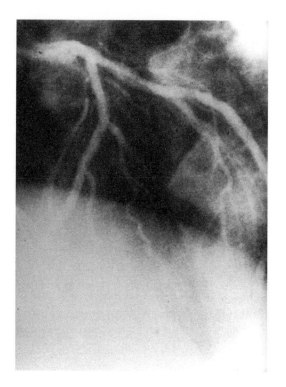

Narrowing of blood vessels by atherosclerosis is one of the commonest causes of cardiac and cerebral disease. These angiograms show (left) severe narrowing of the anterior descending coronary artery and (right) restoration of normal blood flow after angioplasty. In this chapter we discuss the pathology of atherosclerosis and other vascular diseases.

(Reproduced with kind permission from Dr Howard Swanton, UCL Hospitals Trust, London.)

Vascular pathology

■ CONTENTS

Case 11.1

A 61-year-old man was admitted to hospital complaining of pain in the left side of his chest and radiating down his left arm. He also felt nauseated and had vomited twice before arrival. His electrocardiogram (ECG) showed signs of an anterior infarct and chest X-ray showed evidence of heart failure. He was given diamorphine to control his pain and diuretics for his cardiac failure, and admitted to the intensive care unit. The following morning, he had ventricular arrhythmia and cardiac arrest from which he could not be resuscitated.

Postmortem examination revealed extensive atheroma in all major vessels and triple coronary vessel disease. The anterior descending coronary artery showed 90% narrowing along its length together with evidence of recent plaque fissuring and acute thrombosis with complete occlusion. A large anterior infarct was confirmed. Cardiac failure and an old cerebral infarct were also noted.

Cardiovascular disease is the biggest cause of mortality, accounting for approximately 33% of all deaths. The example illustrated above is an all too familiar scenario in hospitals. Fortunately not all patients die so abruptly following a myocardial infarction.

In this chapter, we will examine the various components of the vascular system and then explore the pathological processes that lead to the development of thrombosis and infarction. We will also consider the complications resulting from this process and consider potential therapeutic options for patient management.

THROMBOSIS

A thrombus is a mass composed of blood constituents and results from an interaction between the endothelial cells lining the vessels, the platelets, and the coagulation system. It occurs within a closed cardiovascular system and in this respect it is not quite the same as a clot occurring outside the body.

Thrombosis can be classified as either *arterial* or *venous*. Arterial thrombosis tends to occur in the elderly and in those with peripheral vascular disease, for instance diabetics. Venous thrombosis, in contrast, is generally seen with the immobility that accompanies postoperative bed rest.

The factors important in the development of thrombosis were worked out over 100 years ago by Rudolf Virchow and are known as *Virchow's triad*. He suggested that thrombosis is caused by one or more of the following factors:

- Alteration in the blood constituents.
- Damage to the endothelial cells.
- Changes in the flow of the blood.

In order to understand how these three factors might lead to thrombus formation, it is worthwhile digressing briefly to consider the normal homeostatic mechanisms within the vascular system (also briefly described in Chapter 2).

NORMAL VASCULAR HOMEOSTASIS

If there is damage to the vascular system, for example when you cut yourself with a knife, the normal homeostatic mechanisms come into play in order to stop the bleeding. The three main constituents are the platelets, the vessel wall, and the proteins of the coagulation pathway (Fig. 11.1).

When a vessel is damaged, it constricts ('vasoconstriction'), which slows the flow of blood. The connective tissue of the vessel, which is exposed in the process, attracts platelets to adhere to the site of injury. Platelets release soluble factors which help to lay down fibrin via the coagulation pathway. This stable plug helps to stop the bleeding and hence begins the process of healing. Of course this does not go unchecked. Just as the coagulation system is being activated to produce the fibrin plug, inactivating proteins (fibrinolysins) are also produced to stop the process and to digest the fibrin plug. This results in a complex interaction between positive and negative factors which allows the bleeding to be stopped without the whole vascular system turning into one giant thrombus.

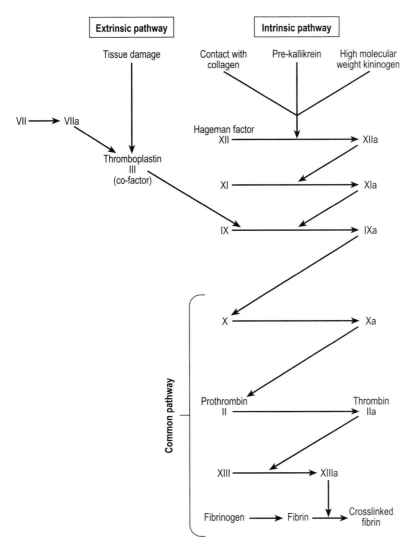

Fig. 11.1 Simplified illustration of the coagulation pathway. Tissue damage or activation of the intrinsic pathway by, for example, contact with collagen activates a series of enzymes that leads to deposition of fibrin, which together with platelets forms a plug to prevent uncontrolled bleeding. When it occurs in a small vessel such as a coronary artery, it leads to obstruction and hence infarction.

Platelets

Platelets are cytoplasmic fragments produced by megakaryocytes in the bone marrow (see Chapter 5). Their role in thrombosis can be divided into three phases, *adhesion*, *secretion*, and *aggregation*. When the vascular endothelium is damaged and collagen is exposed, the first event is adhesion of platelets. This is achieved via receptors on the platelet surface. Following this, the platelets release the contents of their granules. These are needed for the coagulation pathway and also induce platelet aggregation. Secretion from the platelets stimulates the intrinsic pathway of the coagulation cascade (Fig. 11.1), resulting in the production of thrombin. Thrombin acts to stimulate platelets and so enhances the reaction.

Coagulation components

The components involved in the coagulation pathway are shown in Figure 11.1. The final product of this pathway is *fibrin*, which acts to stabilize the plug of aggregated platelets. The coagulation pathway has been divided traditionally into the extrinsic and intrinsic pathways, although a complex interplay occurs between them. The common pathway begins at factor X, which acts on prothrombin to produce thrombin, which itself has a variety of actions but most importantly converts fibrinogen to fibrin (feedback loops and the control mechanisms which inhibit or inactivate reactions have been omitted for simplicity). The most important enzyme capable of digesting fibrin is plasmin. This is produced from plasminogen either by a factor XII-dependent pathway, by therapeutic agents such as streptokinase, or by tissue-derived plasminogen activators (tPA). Conveniently, some plasminogen is bound to fibrin as a thrombus is formed and so is perfectly situated for conversion by the tPA to plasmin, which can then digest the thrombus. Compounds capable of breaking down thrombi have enormous therapeutic potential for restoring blood flow, and both streptokinase and synthetic tPA are used in suspected myocardial infarction.

Endothelium

The endothelium is normally resistant to thrombus formation, which is remarkable, since it is capable of both initiating and terminating thrombosis. Normally these two activities are finely balanced in favour of preventing thrombus formation. Damage to the endothelium, however, tips the balance towards thrombosis. Under normal circumstances, the endothelium prevents the elements of blood from coming into contact with the subendothelial connective tissue (collagen), which is highly thrombogenic. In vessels affected by atheroma, not only is the endothelium more readily damaged but the subendothelial tissue consists of the components of atheroma, which are extremely thrombogenic.

Let us consider how Virchow's triad may apply to clinical situations. In myocardial infarction, the atheroma in the coronary arteries occludes the lumen, resulting in changes in *flow*. It also damages the *endothelium*, resulting in exposure of collagen to the blood, which sets up a thrombotic cascade. This will result in sudden obstruction to the blood flow, leading to ischaemia and infarction of the muscle supplied by the vessel. This is an example of thrombosis occurring in the arterial side of the circulation.

Another example is polycythaemia. In this condition, there is an increase in the number of red cells in the blood, due to either a physiological adaptation (e.g. living at high altitude) or neoplastic proliferation. The increase in blood cells leads to a sluggish *flow* and hence a propensity to thrombus formation. This type of thrombosis is common in the venous side of the circulation.

Hence, while the platelets and coagulation system are designed to protect us from bleeding to death, under some circumstances the process can damage organs and may even be fatal. Let us now assume that a thrombus has occurred in some part of the vascular system. What may happen next?

POSSIBLE OUTCOMES FOLLOWING THROMBOSIS

1. The ideal outcome would be that the system halts the thrombotic process and removes the debris to leave a normal blood vessel. This process is termed *resolution*.
2. If the thrombus cannot be removed, it may be *organized* or *recanalized*.
3. The thrombus may be cast off into the circulation as an *embolus*.

Resolution occurs commonly in the small veins of the lower limb following thrombosis. This is possibly due to the fact that venous intima contains more plasminogen activator than arterial intima. Drugs with a thrombolytic action, such as streptokinase, can be given to patients early after thrombosis to promote dissolution of the clot and hence resolution. The drug has to be given within hours because it has much less effect on polymerized fibrin, which predominates later.

Organization of a thrombus involves similar processes to the organization of inflammation described in Chapter 2. When the thrombus has formed, polymorphs and macrophages begin to degrade and digest the fibrin and cell debris. Later, granulation tissue grows into the base of the thrombus. Ultimately, the thrombus shrinks and is covered by endothelial or smooth muscle cells.

Recanalization is a term used to describe the production of *new* endothelial-lined channels which convey blood through the occlusive thrombus. This is thought to occur by the production of clefts within the thrombus, resulting from a combination of local digestion and shrinkage. The clefts extend through the thrombus and become lined by endothelial cells derived from the adjacent intima.

EMBOLISM

An embolus is a portion of solid, liquid, or gaseous material which is carried in the blood from one area of the circulatory system to another area. The majority of emboli arise from thrombi and the term *thromboembolism* is sometimes used synonymously with embolism. There are many other, though admittedly rarer, causes of emboli. These include:

- Fragments of atheromatous plaques.
- Bone marrow.
- Fat.
- Air or nitrogen.
- Amniotic fluid.
- Tumour.
- Foreign material, e.g. intravenous catheter.

Where emboli lodge depends on their size, origin, and in which side of the circulation they occur. Those arising in the venous side pass through the right side of the heart to the pulmonary circulation (pulmonary emboli). Those that arise in the left side of the circulation will block systemic arteries and the clinical effect will depend on the organ involved, e.g. brain, kidneys, or the periphery of limbs.

Pulmonary embolism

The lungs are unusual organs because they have a dual blood supply. The lung receives deoxygenated blood via the pulmonary arteries and oxygenated blood from bronchial arteries feeding directly from the aorta. Hence, the lungs have an established *collateral* arterial circulation. This means that occlusion of a branch of the pulmonary artery rarely causes infarction of the lung parenchyma (unless the bronchial supply is compromised) and, because the alveolar walls are intact, resolution is possible. The effects of a pulmonary embolus thus depend on the size of the occluded vessel, the number of emboli, and the adequacy of the bronchial blood supply. Obstruction of the main pulmonary artery, however, can have profound effects on the circulation, as can numerous emboli occurring together. Small emboli to peripheral vessels have little effect unless the bronchial supply is compromised by the presence of concomitant cardiac failure. The eventual fate of the embolus is similar to that of a thrombus. It may be removed completely or it may be organized and recanalized.

Systemic embolism

Most of the emboli in the left side of the circulation originate in the heart itself from thrombi forming on areas of myocardial infarction. Other causes include fragments of atheromatous plaques, which arise from fissuring or ulceration of a plaque which releases its fibrin, lipid, and cholesterol mixture into the circulation. Arterial emboli almost always cause infarction. For instance, emboli to the lower limbs may lead to gangrene of the toes. Emboli to the brain cause a 'stroke' (cerebrovascular accident), which may lead to death. A special type of systemic embolus is the infected material from vegetations on the heart valves in infective endocarditis. These produce septic infarcts and abscesses in the affected tissues (Fig. 11.2)

THE PROCESS OF ATHEROSCLEROSIS

Having considered thrombosis and embolism, we will now look at the major cardiovascular problems of later life, namely arteriosclerosis and myocardial infarction. These are overwhelming causes of morbidity and mortality in developed countries, but they are not an inevitable consequence of ageing, and so it is of great importance to try to identify the causative and risk agents.

Let us consider another clinical problem.

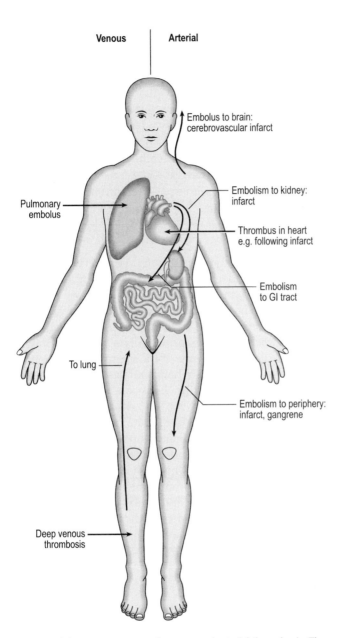

Venous | Arterial

Embolus to brain:
cerebrovascular infarct

Embolism to kidney:
infarct

Pulmonary
embolus

Thrombus in heart
e.g. following infarct

Embolism
to GI tract

To lung

Embolism to periphery:
infarct, gangrene

Deep venous
thrombosis

Fig. 11.2 Illustration of the consequences of venous and arterial thrombosis. The main embolic complications of venous thrombosis are pulmonary emboli. The arterial thrombus may result in emboli to various organs, including brain, kidney, GI tract, and periphery.

Case 11.2

A 52-year-old man complains of blurring of his vision. He has diabetes, a metabolic disorder characterized by hyperglycaemia (raised blood glucose). At the age of 10 years, he presented with the typical diabetic symptoms of tiredness, weight loss, polyuria (increased urine production), and polydypsia (increased thirst). The blood glucose was raised, glucose was found in his urine, and he has been on insulin ever since.

He also complains of shortness of breath, especially on exertion, and cramps in his calf muscles on exercise. On examination, he was found to have a raised blood pressure, with small haemorrhages and small blood vessel proliferation in his retina.

This man has widespread disease related to his arterial system. The arterial pathology comes under the general heading of *arteriosclerosis*, popularly referred to as 'hardening of the arteries'. His large and medium-sized arteries are likely to be narrowed by fibrolipid *atherosclerotic* lesions and his small arteries and arterioles will show the proliferative or hyaline changes of *arteriosclerosis*. *Atherosclerosis* is principally a disease of the intima (inner layer) and may result in narrowing of the vessel, obstruction, or thrombosis. *Arteriolosclerosis*, on the other hand, affects the media (muscle layer), with a resultant increase in wall thickness and decreased elasticity which may lead to hypertension.

Let us examine his symptoms. His diabetes makes him much more likely to develop atherosclerosis. Atheromatous plaques in his coronary arteries will result in chronic ischaemia and cardiac failure. Because the left side of the heart generally fails first this will result in pulmonary oedema and shortness of breath. The combination of poor cardiac function and atheroma in the abdominal aorta and limb vessels explains the pain and cramp in his calf muscle (intermittent claudication). His blurred vision may also be of vascular origin, as the retina is frequently affected by small haemorrhages and new vessel formation.

The atheromatous plaque

The atheromatous plaque is raised above the surrounding intima and protrudes into the lumen. It is whitish-yellow in colour. On sectioning, the plaque is composed of a fibrous cap covering a soft yellow fatty (lipid) centre, which looks like porridge or gruel and is called atheroma. At the edges of the lesion, there may be new vessel formation. The plaques are common in the aorta, femoral, carotid, and coronary arteries, where they may produce symptoms due to occlusion, thrombosis, embolism, or aneurysm formation.

In contrast, hyaline and hyperplastic arteriolosclerotic changes affect small vessels, do not contain lipid, and primarily affect the media (muscle layer), whereas atheroma is initially an *intimal* problem. Hyaline arteriolosclerosis generally occurs in elderly or diabetic patients and involves the deposition of homogeneous, pink material which thickens the media, resulting in a narrowed vessel. Hyperplastic arteriolosclerosis is found in patients who have a sudden or severe prolonged increase in blood pressure. The media of the vessel wall is thickened by a concentric proliferation of smooth muscle cells and an increase in basement membrane material.

Risk factors for atheroma formation

Age

Ischaemic heart disease is common with advancing age. However, it is not an inevitable consequence of ageing. The atheromatous process affects different vessels at different ages. Thus, small aortic lesions may appear as early as the first decade of life, coronary artery lesions in the second decade, and cerebral arterial lesions in the third decade.

Sex

Men are much more likely to die with cardiovascular disease than women. This is related to the protective effect of oestrogens. Myocardial infarction is extremely rare in premenopausal women.

Smoking

Smoking is a significant risk factor for atheroma. One packet of cigarettes a day increases the likelihood of having a myocardial infarction by 300%. Besides an effect on atheroma, smoking also influences local thrombotic tendencies due to altered platelet function. How smoking damages vessels is not known, but suggestions include increased free radical activity, raised carbon monoxide levels, or a direct effect of nicotine.

Hypertension

Hypertension (raised blood pressure) is also a significant risk factor for ischaemic heart disease and cerebrovascular accidents ('strokes'). Drug treatment to reduce the blood pressure reduces the risk in patients with moderate to severe hypertension. The value of drugs in mild hypertension is unclear.

Hyperlipidaemia

Evidence for the role of fats in atheroma has been derived from both experimental and epidemiological studies. There is good evidence that in populations with a high incidence of atherosclerosis, there are high plasma concentrations of certain lipids, namely low density lipoproteins (LDL) rich in cholesterol and very low density lipoproteins (VLDL). In contrast, high density lipoproteins (HDL) appear to be cardioprotective. Note: *high* density means *low* in fat.

Diabetes

As we have discussed in the clinical example, the risk of atheroma is increased in diabetics (see Chapter 10 for why this is). Myocardial infarction is twice as common as in non-diabetic patients.

Other possible risk factors

There are many other potential risk factors, not all of which have been proved beyond doubt to be real. They include lack of regular exercise, obesity, high carbohydrate intake, oral contraceptives, 'type A' personality (the high-pressure business type), and raised uric acid levels and gout.

Complications of atheroma

Plaques in themselves do not cause any symptoms. They cause problems by reducing the size of the lumen of the blood vessel and hence causing ischaemia and infarction. They also act as a focus for the formation of thrombosis by plaque ulceration and hence embolism. By weakening the wall of the vessel they predispose to local dilatation (aneurysm). Haemorrhage may occur within plaques and the resulting haematoma may distend and crack the plaque leading to ulceration and thrombus formation. In almost all advanced cases, there is some degree of dystrophic calcification in the plaques which, if extensive, will turn the artery into a stiff pipe. These complications are summarized in Box 11.1.

The two commonest clinical manifestations of atherosclerosis are myocardial infarction and cerebral infarction. We will now consider myocardial infarction in more detail.

MYOCARDIAL INFARCTION

Look back at the clinical scenario at the beginning of this chapter. Let us consider the pathological process that led to our patient's myocardial infarction and the complications that might have arisen.

In myocardial infarction the cardiac muscle cells die from a lack of nutrients, most importantly oxygen. Generally, this results from total occlusion of one or more coronary arteries. The extent of the damage will depend on the amount of collateral circulation, the metabolic requirements of the cells at the time, and the duration of the ischaemia. By reducing the size of the lumen, atheroma itself may cause clinical symptoms. The patient may complain of chest pain on exercise which is relieved on resting. This is called

---

■ **BOX 11.1 Complications of atheroma**

Narrowing of vascular lumen
Damage to vessel wall leading to aneurysm formation
Plaque fissuring
Plaque haemorrhage
Thrombus formation
Embolism
Ischaemia and infarction
Rupture of vessel
Dissection of vessel wall

angina and occurs because the myocardial cells become ischaemic but, at this stage, the damage is reversible. If the plaque is suddenly complicated by thrombus to produce complete occlusion of a coronary artery, or if the blood flow is insufficient for even a moderate increase in cardiac work, the patient may go on to develop an infarct. How does an inactive atheromatous plaque suddenly occlude a vessel? The fibrous cap of the plaque splits or cracks, letting the blood into the soft necrotic centre. This may distort and enlarge the plaque but, more importantly, it activates the thrombotic cascade. The resulting infarct may involve a variable thickness of the myocardial wall, but when it involves the full thickness of the wall, it is referred to as a *transmural* infarction (Fig. 11.3). 90% of transmural infarctions

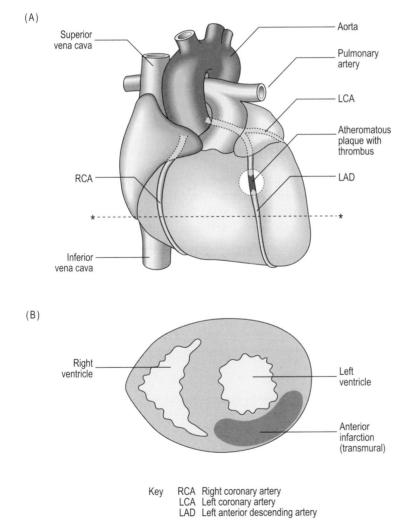

Key   RCA Right coronary artery
LCA Left coronary artery
LAD Left anterior descending artery

Fig. 11.3 (A) Heart and major vessels with an obstruction to the left anterior descending artery (LAD). This will lead to ischaemia and infarction in the region supplied by the vessel. (B) Section of myocardium taken at level shown in (A). This shows an area of transmural (full thickness) infarction involving the anterior and septal parts of the left ventricle.

result from thrombosis complicating atheroma. Myocardial infarction is much more common in the left ventricle and interventricular septum than the right ventricle. *Subendocardial* infarction is much less common than transmural infarction. It is confined to the inner half of the myocardium and may be circumferential. A very thin layer of subendocardial muscle remains viable because it receives nutrients and oxygen from the ventricular luminal blood.

The pathological appearances of myocardial infarction

The ECG showed our patient to have had an anterior infarct. The autopsy revealed a thrombus in the left anterior descending artery. This artery supplies the anterior wall of the left ventricle. No gross abnormality would be seen if he had died within a few hours. If he died more than 24 hours after infarction, the infarcted area would either appear pale or be red-blue owing to the trapped blood. Later the dead myocardium becomes pale yellow, softened and better defined with a rim of hyperaemic (red, congested) tissue at the periphery. Over the next few weeks, the necrotic muscle is replaced by fibrous scar tissue and this is usually complete by 6 weeks. The exact time course depends on the size of the infarct and any complications that may occur.

Complications of myocardial infarction

These are summarized in Box 11.2 and will be of particular interest to those in contact with patients in intensive care. The commonest complications are *cardiac failure* and *arrhythmias*. Arrhythmias are responsible for sudden death following myocardial infarction (as in our example). The arrhythmias occur because of either ischaemia or death of the specialized conduction system of the heart. Cardiac failure may occur because of extensive death of muscle cells in the left ventricular wall. Cardiac failure will also occur if the

---

■ **BOX 11.2 Complications of myocardial infarction**

Cardiac arrhythmias
Cardiac failure
Rupture of papillary muscle with valve prolapse
Pericarditis
Thrombus formation
Emboli from thrombus in ventricle or atria which may cause:
   renal damage
   cerebrovascular accident (stroke)
   infarction of peripheral tissues
Aneurysm of ventricular wall
Rupture of ventricular septum causing ventricular septal defect (VSD)
Rupture of ventricle with bleeding into pericardium leading to tamponade
Death

heart valves do not function properly as a result of the damage sustained during the infarct. The *papillary muscles* which support the valves may be damaged and *rupture*, allowing the valve leaflet to prolapse. Similar softening occurs in infarcted tissue in the left ventricular wall, so that it too may *rupture*. This occurs in transmural infarction (i.e. full thickness) but not in subendocardial infarction. Within 48 hours of transmural infarction, the damaged ventricular muscle stretches and becomes thinner, and is therefore liable to *aneurysm* formation. Rupture of the ventricular wall may lead to blood escaping into the pericardial space (*haemopericardium*), which inhibits the normal action of the heart and leads to *cardiac tamponade*, which is fatal unless treated. The body's immune system responds to the infarction, so that the pericardial surface overlying the damaged area usually becomes inflamed (*pericarditis*) by the second or third day. This may produce a *pericardial rub* which may be heard through a stethoscope. Similar inflammatory changes occur on the endocardial surface of the infarct, which, in combination with stasis, may lead to *intraventricular thrombosis*. Embolism may occur systemically as a further consequence.

CEREBRAL INFARCTION

As mentioned earlier, cerebrovascular infarction (stroke) is another common manifestation of atherosclerosis. There are similarities, in the pathogenesis of stroke and myocardial infarction. In simple terms, a 'stroke' results from a change in the vascular supply of the brain. By analogy with angina in the heart, ischaemia lasting for a short time in the central nervous system is called a *transient ischaemic attack* (TIA). Longer periods of ischaemia result in infarction.

The mechanisms responsible for cerebrovascular accident include thrombosis complicating atheroma in the carotid vessels, emboli arising from the heart and travelling to the brain, heart injury, and subarachnoid haemorrhage which may result from rupture of a berry aneurysm. The clinical manifestations will depend on the site and nature of the lesion. Most 'strokes' occur within the cerebral hemisphere in the region of the middle cerebral artery and result in contralateral hemiparesis (sensory and motor disturbance on the opposite side of the body). The degree of sensory loss and paralysis depends on the size and position of the damaged brain tissue. If the area of infarction is very small, it may not produce any symptoms at all, and occasionally postmortem examination reveals multiple infarcts which were not apparent during life. Such multiple infarcts may contribute to dementia in the elderly.

Pathological features of cerebral infarction

At a very early stage, no pathological changes are visible. After about 24 hours, the affected tissue becomes soft and friable. There is usually oedema of the surrounding tissues. After a few days, the area becomes frankly necrotic and, since the brain contains a lot of fat and water, the tissue takes on the appearance of liquid, hence the term liquefactive necrosis. As the infarct heals and the debris is removed, there is a reaction leading to 'scar' formation. In the brain, this is due to proliferation of glial tissue and is called *gliosis*. If there is bleeding into the infarcted area owing to damage of blood vessels, the infarct is termed *haemorrhagic*.

Complications of cerebral infarction

Complications include reversible and irreversible sensory deficit and paralysis of the opposite side of the body – i.e. a right-sided infarct produces left-sided signs. The disability may involve part (e.g. face only) or the whole of the body. The patient may die immediately or without regaining consciousness if vital structures such as the respiratory centre are damaged. If the infarct involves the left side of the brain, varying degrees of speech malfunction (*aphasia*) may also be present.

Patients who have survived an infarct are still at risk of further events, since the underlying problem is usually severe atheromatous disease or long-standing hypertension.

HYPERTENSION

Hypertension is a significant factor in atheroma formation and it is also a treatable condition. Hence, it offers a target for the prevention of cardiac disease. Hypertension is very common, affecting approximately 25% of adults – on the basis that a blood pressure of greater than 140/90 mmHg is regarded as abnormal. It predominantly affects people in middle and later life, and can be divided into *benign* and *malignant* forms. Fortunately, benign hypertension, which accounts for 95% of the cases, is much more common, is relatively stable, and is treatable with long-term antihypertensive drugs. It may be *primary* (or idiopathic, meaning 'no apparent cause') or *secondary*. Secondary hypertension is generally due to kidney disease, with a small number due to endocrine abnormalities. Malignant hypertension only affects 5% of patients, but it is more severe and is liable to affect men under 50 years of age. The major complications of hypertension are cardiac disease, cerebrovascular accidents, and chronic renal failure. Box 11.3 summarizes these.

■ **BOX 11.3 Complications of hypertension**

Intracerebral haemorrhage from microaneurysms
Cerebrovascular accident (stroke)
Cardiac failure with pulmonary oedema
Left ventricular hypertrophy
Myocardial infarction
Ischaemic renal damage and renal failure
Atherosclerosis and all its complications

There are a large number of antihypertensive drugs available, and with proper control it should be possible to reduce the morbidity and mortality that results from cardiac disease. One problem is that hypertension often goes unnoticed, as it may not produce symptoms until severe cardiac disease is already present. Further, as with any condition that does not produce symptoms but requires long-term treatment, there may be a lack of compliance. Hypertension is also only one element in the predisposition to heart disease, and the patient may require fundamental changes to his lifestyle, including alterations in exercise patterns, diet, stress levels, and smoking.

In summary, vascular diseases and their complications constitute some of the commonest reasons for hospital admission and for autopsy requests (see Appendix 3 for the rules governing autopsy). An understanding of their causes and complications should lead to an understanding of the possible ways to prevent the terrible toll from these disorders.

FURTHER READING

Cooper M W 1988 Cardiology handbook for health professionals. Green, St. Louis, 186 pp

Cotran R S, Kumar V, Robbins S L 1994 Pathological basis of disease, 5th edn. Saunders, Philadelphia, 1400 pp

De Bono D 1990 Practical coronary thrombosis. Blackwell, Oxford 122 pp

Hart J T, Stilwell B, Muir J A 1993 Prevention of coronary heart disease and stroke. Faber & Faber, London, 351 pp

Tutorial 11

Here are some questions to test and extend your knowledge of vascular pathology. They may require some additional 'looking up' in textbooks!

QUESTIONS

1. What do you think is meant by 'disseminated intravascular coagulation' (DIC)?

2. What do you understand by 'shock' in relation to vascular pathology?

3. What is an aneurysm? Give examples of different types.

4. What do you think is meant by 'adult respiratory distress syndrome' (ARDS)?

5. What can be learned about the peripheral vascular system by looking at a patient's limbs?

ANSWERS

1. Disseminated intravascular coagulation results from a loss of proper control in the clotting and fibrinolytic systems. There is no single typical clinical presentation, since any organ may be affected and the major problem may be excessive clotting, which plugs numerous vessels, or inadequate clotting, resulting in uncontrolled haemorrhage. As a general rule, sudden-onset DIC presents with bleeding problems and is particularly associated with obstetrical complications (amniotic fluid emboli). In contrast, chronic DIC is commoner in patients with disseminated cancer and the thrombotic manifestations dominate. The fundamental problem is that there is excessive activation of coagulation, which ultimately is complicated by consumption of the coagulation factors and overactivity of the fibrinolytic system.

2. 'Shock' in the context of vascular pathology means a state of circulatory collapse. The shocked patient will require intensive treatment of the condition which has produced the circulatory collapse and also of the widespread ischaemic damage resulting from it. The blood pressure may or may not be low depending on compensatory mechanisms. What might be the cause? There may be insufficient circulating volume (e.g. due to bleeding, diarrhoea etc.); this is called *hypovolaemic* shock. Abrupt heart failure may result from myocardial infarction, arrhythmias and cardiac tamponade. This is *cardiogenic* shock. A rather special but clinically very important form of shock is '*septic shock*' due to overwhelming infection, especially with Gram-negative bacteria which contain toxic lipopolysaccharides ('endotoxin').

3. An aneurysm is a localized dilatation of the heart muscle or a blood vessel. Examples include cardiac aneurysm following myocardial infarction, berry aneurysms which are due to developmental defects in the cerebral vessels, and syphilitic aneurysms that classically occur in the proximal aorta owing to inflammatory damage following the infection. Atherosclerotic aneurysms, in contrast, occur in the descending abdominal part of the aorta. The main dangers of aneurysms are pressure on adjacent tissues and rupture.

4. ARDS stands for *adult respiratory distress syndrome*. The lungs are resistant to short periods of ischaemia, but if it is prolonged, as in massive trauma, the patient may develop 'shock lung' or ARDS. In ARDS there is severe oedema affecting peribronchial connective tissue and alveolar septae and spaces. This reduces the lung compliance and impairs alveolar diffusion, and carries a mortality rate of around 50%. The damaged alveolar capillary *endothelial* cells are leaky, which leads to interstitial alveolar oedema and fibrin exudation. The damaged alveolar *epithelial* cells desquamate and contribute to the characteristic *hyaline membranes*. These are the same as the hyaline membranes seen in neonatal hyaline membrane disease, and in both situations they indicate severe epithelial injury with lack of surfactant. The lack of surfactant leads to collapse of alveolar air spaces (atelectasis) and so further reduces compliance and gas transfer.

5. Peripheral vascular disease leads to ischaemia of the limbs, and there may be few or numerous clues. These include atrophy of muscles, loss of hair, atrophic shiny skin, cold peripheries, lack of detectable pulses and, in severe cases, frank gangrene of toes or fingers.

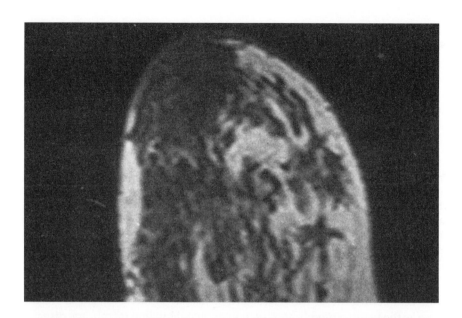

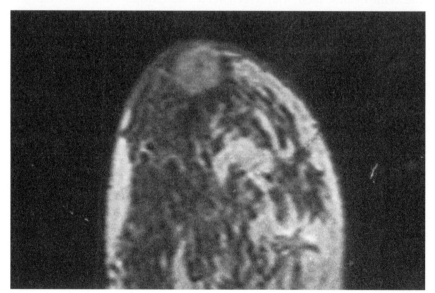

A breast tumour revealed by mammography. Contrast enhancement (by Gadolinium chelate) improves the resolution (compare bottom with top). This is one of the more common tumours, and in this chapter we discuss how tumours are classified, why they form, why some are more serious than others, and the ways in which they can be treated.

(Reproduced with kind permission from Mr Douek and Mr Gafhour, UCL Medical School, London.)

Neoplasia

12

Case 12.1

A 72-year-old retired general practitioner presented to his family doctor with bleeding from the rectum. He was referred to the local hospital where sigmoidoscopy revealed an ulcerated tumour. Biopsy confirmed an adenocarcinoma.

A laparotomy was carried out to resect his bowel cancer. At this time there was no evidence of metastases. The pathological examination revealed a 3 cm tumour which was poorly differentiated and penetrated the full thickness of the bowel wall. Vascular permeation was seen and 4 of 15 lymph nodes contained tumour (Duke's stage C). A number of dysplastic adenomatous polyps were also found adjacent to the tumour.

He represented 1 year later with weight loss and cachexia. At this time, multiple metastases in the liver were identified. He died 6 months later.

Many people reading this book will have come into contact with cancer, either through work or because someone in the family has been directly or indirectly affected. The word cancer produces a fear that is difficult to allay, but is not entirely justified. Although we are all aware that heart disease kills, few of us have the same dread of dying from a myocardial infarction as of dying from cancer. In fact cancer is not one disease but includes more than a hundred different types. Great advances have been made in the management and treatment of certain types such as Hodgkin's disease, leukaemias, and testicular tumours, and even complete cures are now possible.

In this chapter, we will examine the features of malignant neoplasms ('new growths'), the classification of tumours, the causes of cancer including 'cancer genes', how cancers grow and behave, and the treatment(s) available. We will also look briefly at benign neoplasms and how these differ from malignant tumours.

THE FEATURES OF MALIGNANT TUMOURS

These can be divided into clinical and pathological features. Both are important in arriving at a diagnosis of malignancy.

The single most important clinical manifestation of malignancy is *metastasis*. If, in the example considered above, the patient had had enlarged lymph nodes and liver, the diagnosis of malignancy would have been a certainty. Failing that, the physician or surgeon has to rely on a variety of other features. Malignant tumours tend to be larger in *size* than benign ones, although this is not an absolute rule. Owing to their infiltrative pattern, malignant tumours are usually *adherent* to neighbouring tissues, while benign ones are often mobile and move over nearby tissues. Both benign and malignant tumours ulcerate but in the specific situation described above, the ulcerated mass in the rectum favours a carcinoma. Rectal bleeding has to be considered as coming from a malignancy unless proved otherwise. In this case, the tumour has eroded the underlying vasculature, resulting in bleeding into the lumen of the bowel. The presence of dysplastic polyps, which represent precursor lesions, also aids the diagnosis. All these features help to convince the doctor that the lesion is malignant.

The pathologist uses a similar system to assess whether a tumour is benign or malignant. The gross examination of the resection specimen is important as it allows the pathologist to assess some of the features already mentioned. These include the size of the tumour, whether it is ulcerated, how far into the wall it infiltrates, whether it appears to involve adjacent structures, and, most importantly, whether it appears to have been completely excised.

Further information will come from the *histological* examination. Again, the first thing the pathologist has to decide is whether the lesion is benign or malignant. Features that favour malignancy are: disorganized architecture with a loss of the normal polarity of cell arrangement, nuclear pleomorphism (differences in size and shape), hyperchromatism (increased blue staining of nuclei owing to changes in DNA), increased nuclear:cytoplasmic ratio (N:C ratio), and increased numbers of mitoses, especially with abnormal forms (Fig. 12.1). The next question is what type of tumour it is – *primary* (arising locally) or *secondary* (a metastasis). Several things will help with this decision. Does the tumour resemble the normal tissues at that site? Since the colon is composed of glandular tissue, a glandular malignancy (an adenocarcinoma – see classification later) will favour local origin. A squamous carcinoma, on the other hand, would favour a metastasis or extension from an anal carcinoma. Another feature that might help is the presence of *dysplasia* in the adjacent colonic mucosa or within polyps. Severe dysplasia shades into *in situ* carcinoma. A good example is found in the breast, where cells resembling carcinoma are seen within ducts; this is called 'in situ ductal carcinoma', and is believed to represent an earlier stage from which the invasive tumour arises – i.e. it is a precursor lesion. The presence of dysplastic polyps, as in our example, is another clue that the tumour has originated locally. The 'typing' of the tumour is also important from the prognostic point of view. Some organs such as the breast have many different types of locally arising tumours. These include ductal,

Benign

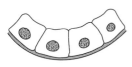

Malignant

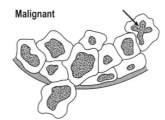

- Polar arrangement of cells with regular architecture
- Small regular nuclei
- Low nuclear:cytoplasmic (N:C) ratio
- Low mitotic count

- Loss of normal polarity with disorganised architecture
- Pleomorphic nuclei (differences in size and shape)
- High nuclear:cytoplasmic (N:C) ratio
- High mitotic count with abnormal forms (arrow)

Fig. 12.1 A comparison of features helpful in distinguishing benign from malignant lesions.

lobular, medullary, and tubular carcinomas, to name only a few. Medullary and tubular carcinomas have been shown to have a better prognosis than ordinary ductal carcinomas, which is clearly useful in the further management of the patient.

Having decided on the type, the pathologist must decide how closely it resembles normal tissue – i.e. the degree of *differentiation*. A well-differentiated tumour closely resembles normal tissue, while a poorly differentiated tumour does not. Sometimes it is not possible to make out any resemblance at all, in which case we speak of *anaplastic* carcinoma. The differentiation and proliferative activity (e.g. number of mitoses) allows the determination of the tumour *grade*. The pathologist will also examine how far the tumour is infiltrating and whether it involves the lymph nodes. This dictates the pathological *stage* of the tumour (our patient's rectal tumour was stage C). Besides the grade and stage, the pathologist can also provide other prognostic information, such as the presence or absence of vascular infiltration by the tumour. Hence the pathologist's examination can help his clinical colleagues to decide on further management. There is a useful shorthand for staging which applies to all cancers, known as the TNM classification. T stands for tumour size, N for nodal status, and M for metastasis. Thus, for a breast cancer, T1 N0 M0 would indicate a tumour of less than 2 cm, without axillary lymph node or distant spread.

THE CLASSIFICATION OF TUMOURS

Table 12.1 illustrates the classification of tumours. You will see that there are three main groups: tumours of epithelia (carcinomas), tumours of connective tissue (sarcomas), and others (specialized tissue tumours, e.g. brain tumours). This classification has evolved over many years and can appear confusing, since some tumours still carry the name of the eminent people who described them rather than the nomenclature illustrated in the table. Also, although the classification was initially based on *histogenesis* (i.e.

Table 12.1 Classification of tumours

Tissue	Benign tumour	Malignant tumour
Epithelium		
Squamous	Squamous papilloma	Squamous cell carcinoma
Glandular	Adenoma	Adenocarcinoma
Transitional	Transitional cell papilloma	Transitional cell carcinoma
Connective tissue		
Fibrous	Fibroma	Fibrosarcoma
Smooth muscle	Leiomyoma	Leiomyosarcoma
Striated muscle	Rhabdomyoma	Rhabdomyosarcoma
Fat	Lipoma	Liposarcoma
Cartilage	Chondroma	Chondrosarcoma
Bone	Osteoma	Osteosarcoma
Others		
Melanocytes	Benign melanocytic naevus	Melanoma
Germ cells	Benign teratoma	Malignant teratoma
		Seminoma
Central nervous system		Glioma
		Oligodendroglioma, etc.
Placenta	Hydatidiform mole	Choriocarcinoma
Lymphoid cells		Lymphoma
Myeloid cells		Leukaemia
Plasma cells	Plasmacytoma	Myeloma

tissue origin), in reality it is based on *differentiation*. For example, the normal epithelium of the bladder is transitional, hence tumours of the bladder are transitional cell carcinomas. But when the transitional epithelium undergoes metaplasia (see Chapter 9) to become squamous, there is the possibility of developing tumours with squamous cell differentiation. Should this be called transitional cell carcinoma (since the original epithelium was transitional) or squamous cell carcinoma? The answer is the latter. It is better to describe what you see than guess at where it originally came from, since in some circumstances it is impossible to tell the tissue of origin.

WHAT CAUSES CANCER?

The prevailing view is that cancer is a disease of genetic material. This is based on evidence from a number of sources. Some cancers have an obvious heritable component; examples include familial retinoblastoma (see later) and familial adenomatous polyposis. This heredity can only be transferred via genetic material (DNA). Genetic analysis has identified chromosomal abnormalities in tumours, and in some cases consistent changes are seen – e.g. the 8:14 translocation in Burkitt's lymphoma. A number of rare inherited disorders involve an inability to repair damaged DNA. One example is xeroderma pigmentosum, and patients with this disorder have an increased susceptibility to skin cancer following damage to DNA by UV light, suggesting that tumours arise from problems with DNA. Finally, DNA recombinant technology has demonstrated that when DNA is taken from tumour cells and transferred into a normal cell, it can carry its malignant characteristics with it. The identification of genes with a direct role in tumour formation (oncogenes) has firmly established cancer as a disease of genes.

Let us now consider the many predisposing and aetiological factors that lead to tumour formation. Although these factors must alter either the structure or the function of DNA in some way, how they do it is not always known.

Age

The incidence of many tumours (e.g. colon, lung, prostate, bronchus) increases with age. However, other tumours (e.g. leukaemias) also occur in children. It is suggested that carcinogens may have an additive effect over time, which may explain the increased incidence with age, but the exact mechanisms remain unclear.

Genetic factors

There are several types of tumour where the risk is higher in close family members, though the increase cannot be precisely specified. Tumour development is not inevitable and other factors such as environmental and dietary influences may modify the risk.

In some tumours, the genetic susceptibility is better understood. In retinoblastoma, for example, it involves loss of a tumour suppressor gene (see later). Retinoblastoma is a malignant tumour of the eye which is commonest in children, 25–30% of cases being hereditary.

Environmental, geographical, and racial factors

These can be very difficult to dissect out separately. For example, a geographical factor may simply be an environmental factor affecting the population of a particular area, such as a sunny climate, radioactive rock formations, or a carcinogen in the water supply. Melanomas in white-skinned Australians occur because of a *racial predisposition*, because they do not have sufficient skin pigmentation to protect them from ultraviolet light, plus the *geographical factor* of a sunny climate. If the Australian emigrates at birth to a cold cloudy land, the risk of melanoma drops significantly.

Numerous environmental agents have been implicated in causing cancer. Smoking is a prime example, and there is a strong association between smoking and lung cancer. This may affect not only the smoker but also the non-smoker who inhales exhaled tobacco smoke (passive smoking). Asbestos exposure increases the risk of developing lung carcinoma and malignant mesothelioma of the pleura and peritoneum. Exposure to β-napthylamine, e.g. in the rubber and dye industries, increases the risk of transitional cell tumours of the bladder. The first example of an environmental cancer was described by Percival Pott, who observed that chimney sweeps had a very high incidence of scrotal cancer, and correctly deduced that this was due to chronic contact with soot.

Carcinogenic agents

There are three major groups of agents involved in carcinogenesis: chemical carcinogens, radiation and viruses.

Table 12.2 lists some examples of chemical carcinogens and the associated tumour sites. They are thought to act by damaging DNA either directly or indirectly after conversion to more toxic chemicals within the body.

Radiation causes chromosomal breakage, translocations, and mutations. Various protein molecules are also damaged. The carcinogenic effect depends on the type and strength of the radiation and the length of exposure, which is why exposure to diagnostic X-rays is kept to a minimum. Some tissues, such as bone marrow, are especially sensitive, and children appear to be more susceptible than adults. Ultraviolet light is important too, since sun exposure is known to cause skin cancers, in particular melanoma, squamous cell carcinoma, and basal cell carcinoma.

Table 12.3 lists some of the viruses causing cancer. Epstein-Barr virus (EBV) is a member of the herpes family. It usually causes infectious mononucleosis (glandular fever or 'kissing disease'). It has a role in two types of cancer – Burkitt's lymphoma and nasopharyngeal carcinoma. It is of interest that the African regions where Burkitt's lymphoma is common are also regions where malaria is endemic. It is thought that malaria causes a degree of immunodeficiency that allows the EBV-infected B lymphocytes to proliferate, with an increased risk of mutation. Burkitt's lymphoma exhibits a specific mutation in the form of 8:14 translocation. The human

Table 12.2 Chemical carcinogens

Example	Cancer	People exposed
Aflatoxin	Liver	All – eating contaminated foodstuff
Arsenic	Skin, lung	Farmers – insecticide spraying
Benzene	Leukaemia	Dye users, rubber industry
Formaldehyde	Nose	Laboratory workers
Hair dyes	Bladder	Hairdressers
Mineral oils	Skin	Metal machiners
Soot	Skin	Chimney sweeps, firefighters

Table 12.3 Viruses and cancer

Virus	Cancer
Hepatitis B	Liver cancer
Human papilloma (HPV) 16,18	Cervical cancer
Human papilloma (HPV) 5	Skin cancer
Epstein-Barr (EBV)	Burkitt's lymphoma
	Nasopharyngeal carcinoma
HTLV1	Adult T cell leukaemia/lymphoma

papilloma virus (HPV) is known to be associated with skin papillomas (warts). HPV is not a single virus but a group of around 50 genetically distinct viruses. Some types appear to produce benign tumours, while others predispose to malignancy. HPV 16 and 18 are implicated in squamous cell carcinoma of the uterine cervix, while HPV 6 and 11 are common in benign lesions. It is not known how HPV alters the cells. HPV is transmitted by sexual intercourse and there is a high incidence of carcinoma of the cervix in those who begin sexual activity at an early age and in those who are promiscuous. Hepatitis B virus (HBV) causes acute and chronic hepatitis, cirrhosis, and carcinoma of the liver. In South-East Asia, where infection with HBV is endemic, the infection is transmitted from mother to child during pregnancy. These children tend to have chronic HBV infection and a high incidence of hepatocellular carcinoma. Since it is now possible to immunize against HBV, this is one example of a preventable tumour. Liver cell carcinomas are also associated with alcoholic liver disease, androgenic steroids, and aflatoxins. Aflatoxins are toxic metabolites of a fungus, *Aspergillus flavus*, which can contaminate food in the tropics. Aflatoxin B is thought to contribute to cancer formation by causing damage to the liver, which perhaps makes it more susceptible to further cellular changes by HBV.

CANCER-CAUSING GENES (ONCOGENES)

The term *oncogene* refers to any gene that carries mutations and directly contributes to neoplastic transformation of the cell. Two major types of oncogenes have been characterized: dominant oncogenes and tumour suppressor genes.

The function of some normal genes is enhanced by mutations, which are therefore referred to as 'activating' or 'gain-in-function' mutations. These genes are also known as 'dominant' oncogenes, since mutation of one allele is sufficient to exert an effect, despite the presence of the normal gene product from the remaining allele. Dominant oncogenes act as *growth factors* or growth factor *receptors* and also play a role in cell signalling and transcription control within the nucleus. In contrast, *tumour suppressor genes* (TSG) are normal genes whose function has been inactivated by mutation, so they are known as 'inactivating' or 'loss-of-function' mutations, and also as 'recessive' oncogenes, since inactivation of both alleles is required to have any effect at the cellular level. They may also exert their effects at the level of the nucleus in terms of both transcription control and control of the cell cycle during mitosis and proliferation. Although 'oncogene' refers to any cancer-causing gene, in practice the term is reserved for the dominant type and special terms (e.g. tumour suppressor genes) are used for the other kinds. Examples of both types are shown in Table 12.4.

There are a number of ways by which the function of oncogenes can be induced, including (1) point mutations, (2) amplification, (3) gene rearrangement/translocation, and (4) deletion of part or whole of a chromosome. Since most of these mechanisms described apply to both types of oncogene, we will consider them together.

Table 12.4 Genes and cancer

Gene type	Tumour type(s)
Oncogenes	
CerbB2	Breast, salivary gland, ovary
N-*ras*	Leukaemia
Ki-*ras*	Lung, ovary, colon
C-*myc*	Leukaemia, lung
Bcl-2	B-cell lymphoma
Tumour suppressor genes	
APC	Colon, stomach
RB	Retinoblastoma, bone, breast
TP53	Breast, colon, and wide range of tumours
NF1 and 2	Neurofibromatosis

Point mutation

This results in the substitution of one base pair in the DNA by another – e.g. of G:C by A:T. Depending on its position, it may cause alteration of the protein structure by changing the amino acid composition or insert a stop signal which will cause the synthesis of the protein molecule to be terminated prematurely. The clearest examples of point mutation in human tumours are found in the *ras* family of genes. *ras* mutations are encountered in both benign and malignant neoplasms.

Gene rearrangement and translocation

This refers to the production of a hybrid chromosome by the joining of part of one chromosome to another. The resulting rearrangement of DNA sequences can lead to the creation of an altered gene (and therefore protein) either by structural change in the gene or by a change in the control of its transcription. Examples include the 8:14 (or 8:22, 2:8) translocation in Burkitt's lymphoma and the 9:22 translocation in chronic myeloid leukaemia (CML).

Amplification

The normal genome contains two 'allelic' copies of each gene. In amplification, one copy is multiplied numerous times, resulting in increased levels of m-RNA and hence of the corresponding protein. Most classes of oncogene have been shown to be amplified in human malignancy. Examples include the N-*myc* oncogene in neuroblastoma and *Cerb*B2 in breast cancer. Only some of these amplifications have been shown to have pathological significance. N-*myc* amplification is correlated with advanced-stage and recurrent neuroblastoma, and *Cerb*B2 amplification in breast cancer correlates with poor prognosis.

Deletion

This ranges from the loss of single base pairs to the loss of entire chromosomes. The small intragenic (within the gene) deletions have similar effects (abnormal protein, stop codons) to point mutations. Larger deletions will of course lead to inactivation of many genes at a time.

THE MULTISTEP THEORY OF NEOPLASIA

The multistep model of carcinogenesis suggests that cancers arise owing to an accumulation of damage in the DNA, rather than from a single insult or 'hit' to the cell. The genetic damage is in the form of both activation of dominant oncogenes and inactivation of tumour suppressor genes. Hence there is both increased proliferation and a loss of growth inhibitory control. Another important set of genes is those involved in normal tissue homeostasis (these are the genes for cell death by apoptosis; see Chapter 2). Damage to these genes leads to an accumulation of cells with damaged DNA, which would normally have committed suicide, resulting in their survival and an increased risk of proliferation. Hence tumours appear to arise when a number of factors come together within the same cell.

A well-studied example of such a model is the colorectal carcinoma. Within the colon there is a well developed and grossly visible precursor lesion in the form of an adenoma, and genetic analysis has been fruitful in demonstrating the accumulation of damage to the DNA in the transition from normal to adenoma and carcinoma, as illustrated in Figure 12.2.

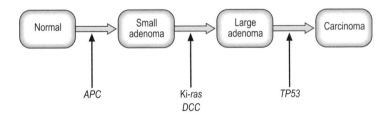

Key *APC* (adenomatous polyposis coli gene)
   DCC (deleted in colon cancer gene)

   APC, DCC and *TP53* are tumour suppressor genes.
   Ki-*ras* is a dominant oncogene.

Fig. 12.2 Hypothetical model illustrating the transition of normal colonic epithelium to adenoma and carcinoma. Alterations in both oncogenes and tumour suppressor genes play a role in the evolution of colon cancer.

FAMILIAL PREDISPOSITION TO CANCER

A number of genes have recently been identified that explain the familial predisposition to malignancy (Table 12.5). The retinoblastoma gene (*RB1*) leads to development of retinoblastoma – a paediatric tumour of the retina. Children inherit one defective copy of the gene from their parent. A subsequent mutation in the second copy of the gene during life leads to tumour formation. Since every retinal cell (and, in fact, every cell in the body!) already has one defective copy, there is a high chance that one retinal cell will get a mutation in the second allele. These tumours occur early in childhood and are often bilateral. Sporadic retinoblastomas also occur, but of course the chances of getting two mutations in the same cell during life, when all the retinal cells start off as normal, are not as high, so sporadic tumours are less common, occur at a later age, and are unilateral. Similarly, the predisposition genes for breast cancer (*BRCA1*, *BRCA2*) have been identified; these genes also predispose to ovarian and male breast cancer. It is worth remembering that the majority of cancers seen in the clinic are due to mutations occurring during the patient's lifetime, and familial predisposition is responsible for only a small minority. For instance, in breast cancer, only 5% of the tumours are due to inherited predisposition and 95% are non-familial. Identification of genes involved in familial predisposition is nevertheless important, because it offers the prospect of genetic counselling in this small group of patients.

These familial predisposition genes are generally tumour suppressor genes and not dominant oncogenes, presumably because mutations in dominant genes are not compatible with normal development of the embryo.

Having discussed how and why tumours occur, let us consider the question that will be at the forefront of the patient's mind: how they behave.

HOW WILL IT BEHAVE?

The behaviour of a tumour is dependent on how fast it will grow, whether it is likely to metastasize, which sites are affected, and what complications result.

It is often assumed that tumours proliferate faster than normal tissues, but this is not necessarily the case. What matters is that there is an *imbalance* between cell production and loss. The time taken for tumour cell division

Table 12.5 Familial predisposition to cancer

Familial syndrome implicated	Cancer(s)	Gene
Hereditary breast and ovary	Breast, ovary	*BRCA1*
Hereditary breast	Breast (male and female)	*BRCA2*
Li-Fraumeni syndrome	Breast, sarcomas	*TP53*
Multiple endocrine neoplasia (MEN syndrome)	Thyroid, adrenal	*RET* [1]
Familial melanoma	Melanoma, pancreas	*p16*

[1]*RET is a dominant oncogene, all the others are tumour suppressor genes.*

varies between 20 and 60 hours, leukaemias having shorter cell cycles than solid tumours, and in general tumour cells take *longer* to divide than their normal counterparts. Some normal tissues, such as the intestine, have a high turnover of cells, with up to 16% of the cells in the growth phase. In contrast, most tumours have only 2–8% of their cells actively dividing. This is important therapeutically because the cells in the growth phase are most readily damaged by chemotherapy, and so tumours with a large growth fraction (e.g. leukaemias, lymphomas, and lung anaplastic small cell carcinoma) will respond better than tumours with few proliferating cells (e.g. colon and breast).

It would also be wrong to assume that every cell in a tumour behaves the same. The cells of an individual tumour are a *clone*, i.e. they are all derived from one parent cell. However, there is genetic evolution in the tumour which results in the production of subclones that may have certain survival advantages; for example, they may have enhanced invasive or metastatic capabilities. This is referred to as *tumour heterogeneity*, and it is important to consider this when planning treatments, because it means that, even within the same patient, tumour cells may respond differently to a given treatment. This is rather analogous to bacterial resistance to antibiotics. Just as a combination of antibiotics may be needed to reduce the chance of selecting out resistant organisms, a mixture of drugs or treatments may have to be used to eradicate all the tumour cells.

The spread of tumours

Over a hundred years ago, Stephen Paget put forward his 'seed and soil' theory of how tumours spread. When you scatter seeds in a field, some of them may grow while others may fail to take hold. He used this analogy to suggest that unless the tumour cells find the right 'soil' they will not grow. An alternative view put forward by James Ewing was that metastases occurred at certain sites owing to the routes of blood supply from the organ of origin. Thus blood from the colon goes to the liver, and this is a common site for metastases. We now know that both theories are true to some extent. Tumours of the colon do indeed go to the liver, but then so do many other tumours from much farther away, such as melanomas arising in the eye. We also know that organs such as the heart and skeletal muscle, despite being exposed to large volumes of blood, rarely contain metastases.

In general, tumour spread through lymphatics will produce metastases in the anatomically related lymph nodes, whilst spread through the blood is influenced more by 'seed and soil' considerations.

Routes of spread

The main routes of spread are via:

- Lymphatics.
- Veins.
- Transcoelomic cavities (pleura, peritoneum, etc.).
- Cerebrospinal fluid.
- Arteries.

Lymphatic spread is common in carcinomas (epithelial tumours), while venous spread is a favoured route for sarcomas (tumours of connective tissues). Arteries are not often penetrated by tumours owing to their muscular wall, except in the later stages of metastatic spread. It is easy to understand how tumours in the pleural or peritoneal cavities can drop into the fluid and be disseminated throughout that cavity. Similarly, the CSF provides a route of spread for cerebral tumours, which do not generally metastasize outside the nervous system.

Metastasis

Let us now consider the steps required to produce a metastasis (Fig. 12.3). First, the tumour has to grow at the site of origin and infiltrate the

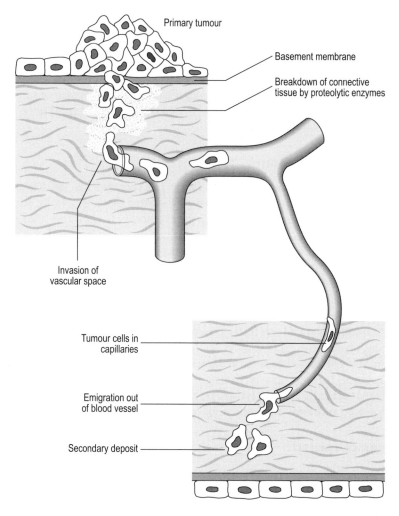

Fig. 12.3 The process of metastasis. The tumour cells have to break through the basement membrane at the site of origin, invade connective tissue, permeate the vascular space, evade the immune system while in the vessel, and emigrate at the end-organ site to form tissue deposit. An incredible journey!

surrounding connective tissue, which may necessitate breaking through a basement membrane by secreting proteolytic enzymes. Then it can reach the lymphatic and blood vascular channels, which are an important route for spread. The vessel wall is traversed and the tumour cells must then detach to float off in the blood or lymph, evading any immune cells (natural killer cells, macrophages, T cells) which might destroy them. Next they must lodge in the capillaries at their destination, attach to the endothelium, and penetrate the vessel wall to enter the perivascular connective tissue, where they finally proliferate to produce a new tumour deposit, or colony. It is a difficult journey for the tumour cells, with many obstacles en route. Tumour metastasis is therefore not a passive but an active, complex process which requires specific properties on the part of the cells. The genetic mechanisms behind these capabilities are being investigated in the hope of interfering with the process therapeutically.

THE CLINICAL EFFECTS OF TUMOURS

The effects of a tumour can be local or systemic.

Local effects

The local effects depend on the site, the type, and the growth pattern of the tumour. Some complications, such as haemorrhage, are more common in malignant tumours because of their ability to invade underlying tissues and blood vessels. Local effects can complicate both benign and malignant tumours. They include:

- Compression of adjacent tissues, e.g. brain tumour compressing nerves and vital structures.
- Obstruction of lumen, e.g. colon or oesophageal tumours.
- Ulceration, e.g. of skin or gastrointestinal tumours.
- Haemorrhage due to erosion of vessels.
- Rupture from obstruction leading to raised pressure, e.g. in the bowel.
- Perforation of tubular structures such as the colon.
- Infarction resulting from damage or obstruction to blood supply.

Systemic effects

A common example is secretion of hormones by an endocrine tumour. Pituitary tumours may produce excess adrenocorticotrophic hormone (ACTH), which will result in Cushing's syndrome. Some non-endocrine tumours can produce hormones 'inappropriately'. One of the commonest examples is in Cushing's syndrome resulting from ACTH produced by oat cell (anaplastic small cell) carcinoma of the bronchus, carcinoid tumours, thymomas, or medullary carcinomas of the thyroid.

Paraneoplastic syndromes are symptoms in cancer patients that are not readily explained by local or metastatic disease. Endocrine effects are generally considered as paraneoplastic if the production is inappropriate (as above), but not if the tumour arises from a tissue that normally produces that hormone. Hypercalcaemia (raised plasma calcium) is an example of paraneoplastic syndrome and is a common and clinically important problem. In a patient with widespread metastases in bone, it may be explained as a local destructive effect of the tumour on bone, which releases calcium. However, hypercalcaemia can occur without metastatic bony deposits and, in some cases, it appears that a parathyroid hormone-like peptide is secreted by the primary tumour. Clubbing of the fingers and hypertrophic osteoarthropathy are also common manifestations of lung carcinoma, though they also occur in non-neoplastic conditions including cyanotic heart disease and liver disease. It is not clear how they develop, nor why sectioning the vagus nerve can lead to their disappearance! Equally mysterious are the skin disorders, peripheral neuropathy, and cerebellar degeneration which may occur in lung carcinoma.

Some general effects of tumours are not classed as paraneoplastic, although they are extremely common and important. These include general malaise, weight loss, and lethargy, which are due to a combination of metabolic and hormonal influences exacerbated by any malnutrition or infection. An important chemical factor that may play a role in weight loss is 'cachexin' – an old name for the cytokine tumour necrosis factor (TNF; see Chapter 5). This molecule is not produced by the tumour cells, but by overactivated macrophages. Anaemia is also common in cancer and can contribute to the general feeling of illness. It may be a direct effect of metastatic deposits in bone marrow or an indirect effect of mediators which suppress haemopoiesis.

TREATMENT OF CANCER

The treatment options available include local excision, radiotherapy, chemotherapy, and palliative treatment. Most patients receive a combination of these, and decisions are based on type of tumour, grading, staging, and individual preferences. Obviously it is not possible to excise a leukaemia, so here chemotherapy has to be the treatment of choice. A breast tumour, however, can be excised but further radiotherapy may be given to prevent recurrence.

Local excision

Local surgery may be aimed at a cure, or simply relief of symptoms. Cancers such as squamous and basal cell carcinomas of the skin and small cancers arising within the ducts in the breast can be cured by local excision. In tumours of the bowel, local excision may relieve an obstruction and provide good long-term remission of symptoms.

Radiotherapy

Radiotherapy aims to kill the cancer cells, but may also damage normal tissues. It is also worth remembering that radiation can actually cause cancer, and this treatment requires careful evaluation of the dose and method of delivery so as not to cause more harm than benefit to the patient. Sometimes an implant can be inserted to provide very localized and specific treatment and minimize toxicity to nearby structures.

Chemotherapy

In patients suffering from haematological malignancies (e.g. leukaemia) or disseminated disease, surgery and radiation are not realistic options. As mentioned above, you cannot excise a leukaemia and you cannot irradiate every single metastasis in the body!

In the 1950s, alkylating agents (e.g. busulphan) and anti-metabolites (e.g. methotrexate) were introduced and proved useful in the management of these disseminated cancers. The main problem is that all of the body's normal tissues are also exposed to the drug, and so the challenge is to deliver enough drug to kill the tumour without killing the patient.

Endocrine-based treatment

Some organs, such as breast and prostate, are hormone-sensitive. Breast carcinomas have receptors for oestrogen which stimulate tumour growth. A drug such as tamoxifen, which acts as an anti-oestrogen, blocks these receptors and reduces progression of the disease. An alternative approach would be to remove the ovaries which produce oestrogen, much as the testes can be removed in males with prostatic adenocarcinoma to reduce the stimulus for tumour growth from androgens.

Immunotherapy

Recombinant DNA technology has enabled the production of cytokines in sufficient quantities for therapeutic use. The *interferons* (IFN) and *tumour necrosis factors* (TNF) are of particular interest. Some tumours, particularly haematological malignancies, have shown dramatic effects with such treatment, while others such as melanomas have been disappointing. Since most tumour cells do not appear to bear specific antigens, trials to increase specific immunity have been rather disappointing. Nevertheless, there is a degree of optimism about a 'cancer vaccine' for certain tumours. In addition, there is considerable interest in raising *monoclonal antibodies* to tumour cells. The hope is that it might be possible to attach drugs or radioisotopes to these antibodies so that they would be delivered specifically to the tumour cell: the concept of the 'magic bullet'. Monoclonal antibodies can also be used in a similar way to 'image' tumours.

Palliative treatment

The treatment of cancer has a broader role than providing a cure. Palliative treatment does not refer to treatment that is given to patients in order to make them comfortable prior to death. It is part of the oncological support given to all cancer patients, and includes not only medication for the control of pain and nausea but also chemotherapy and radiotherapy for the relief of local symptoms.

Fortunately not all tumours are malignant and, in the remainder of the chapter, we will briefly discuss benign tumours and the concept of dysplasia.

BENIGN TUMOURS

The classification in Table 12.1 gives both the benign and malignant counterparts for tumours arising at different sites. Tumours are considered benign when they do not metastasize. Other features that are important in this diagnosis include circumscription (as opposed to invasiveness), smaller size (by no means an absolute feature), lack of pain, little pleomorphism (i.e. monotonous as opposed to 'wild-looking' microscopic appearance), and very few mitoses, without abnormal forms (the opposite being true for malignant tumours). These features are summarized in Table 12.6.

An important point, very often forgotten, is that in certain circumstances the designation of benign and malignant is of minor importance. This is illustrated very well by brain tumours. A glioma, which may be very aggressive and malignant, can certainly kill you. However, a meningioma, which by all the above criteria is benign, may be equally fatal. Since the skull is a closed cavity, even a benign growth will cause a rise in pressure and squeeze the surrounding brain, leading to death unless it is removed. In this situation, the site is of more importance than whether it is benign or malignant.

DYSPLASIA

The term dysplasia was originally used to mean an abnormality of development, but unfortunately it has been misused in the medical literature for a long time. Essentially it describes a set of cytological and architectural abnormalities of tissues with implications for the risk of subsequently developing cancer A familiar example is cervical dysplasia. Dysplasia in the cervical squamous epithelium involves an increased cell size, nuclear pleomorphism, hyperchromatism, loss of orientation of the cells so that they are arranged rather haphazardly, and abnormally sited mitotic activity. These appearances are the same as those described in malignant change, differing only in extent. On the basis of the 'multistep' model of cancer described earlier, it is assumed that if abnormalities can be diagnosed early, then it is possible to treat the 'tumour' at a stage when it is still developing, and hence to cure it. The cervical screening programme aims to pick up the

Table 12.6 Benign versus malignant

Features	Benign	Malignant
Size	Generally small	Often large
Growth	Slow	Fast
Haemorrhage and necrosis	Unusual	Common
Ulceration	Unusual	Common
Tumour margin	Well-circumscribed	Infiltrative
Cell size and shape	Uniform	Pleomorphic
Differentiation	Good	Good to poor
Mitoses	Few – normal forms	Abundant – abnormal forms
Vascular invasion	Absent	May be present
Metastasis	No	Common

abnormalities at the stage of 'dysplasia' or 'pre-cancer'. If even severe dys-plasia is treated, it cannot go on to become an invasive cervical carcinoma. This approach certainly appears to work to a degree. The problem is that we do not have a clear enough picture of the natural history of all grades of dysplasia, and many mild abnormalities almost certainly regress on their own. Predicting which ones will go on to cancer and which will not is far from straightforward, so it is not easy to decide who to treat and who to leave alone.

FURTHER READING

Boon T 1993 Teaching the immune system to fight cancer. Scientific American, March, pp 32–39

Neal A, Hoskins P 1994 Clinical oncology. A textbook for students. Arnold, London, 315 pp

Tjian R 1995 Molecular machines that control genes. Scientific American, February, pp 36–45

What you need to know about cancer. Scientific American (special issue), September 1996

Tutorial 12

Some questions on important issues in the cancer field. None of these can be regarded as 'small print'!

QUESTIONS

1. What is a fibroadenoma of the breast? In what respects does it resemble or differ from a breast carcinoma?

2. What is the role of diet in cancer?

3. Discuss the ways in which cancer can be prevented.

4. What is meant by grade and stage of tumour? Why is it useful to know?

ANSWERS

1. A fibroadenoma is a benign tumour of the breast. It is usually small, round, well circumscribed, and mobile within the breast (its other name – because it moves around in the breast if pushed – is 'breast mouse'). In this respect it is very different from a carcinoma, which by infiltrating surrounding tissues becomes fixed and immobile. Fibroadenomas do not metastasize as carcinomas do. Thus they are similar in that they are both abnormal growths, but the genetic abnormalities of the fibroadenoma do not appear to give it the capacity to invade and kill.

2. This is a very difficult question. Epidemiological studies have been carried out on the association between cancer and various dietary factors, including fibre, fats, and vitamins. They all suffer from the problem that in humans it is hard to look at one factor in isolation. This can be achieved in animal models, but of course they may not be representative of human disease.

Fibre is thought to be protective for colon cancer, while fats (particularly animal fats) are bad and may be implicated in colon and rectal cancer. The data relating to fat in breast cancer are more dubious. What may be even more important are the things that are missing from the diet. Green vegetables and vitamins (e.g. vitamin C) are thought to be protective owing to the antioxidants in these foods which block the effect of free radicals. If you are interested in the question of diet and cancer, there are libraries full of papers on this subject!

3. Bilateral mastectomy or oophorectomy immediately after bearing children would be highly effective but highly impractical! Changes in social habits are more feasible: sunbathing to the extent that you burn leads to skin cancer, particularly melanomas, which can be dramatically reduced by simple avoidance. Giving up smoking can have a dramatic impact on lung cancer. Screening programmes (e.g. cervical) are expensive but have been shown to be effective. The breast screening programme in the UK is predicted to reduce mortality from breast cancer by 25–35%. Can you think of any other ways?

4. Grade is a measure of the *differentiation* of the tumour. In other words, it tells you how closely the tumour resembles the normal tissue from which it arose. Some grading systems, for example for the breast, also incorporate data on proliferation (mitotic count) into the grading system. Its usefulness stems from the fact that many studies (for many different tumour types) have demonstrated that grade is an independent prognostic factor – i.e. the worse the grade, the worse the outlook for the patient.

Stage is a measure of the *extent* of disease. The overall stage is a combination of pathological, radiological, and clinical data. The pathological stage is related to size of tumour and local lymph node metastases. The patients may also have distant metastases which may be identified by radiological techniques such as ultrasound or MRI (magnetic resonance imaging). Again this provides prognostic information, since patients with widespread disease are likely to do worse than patients with localized, non-metastatic disease.

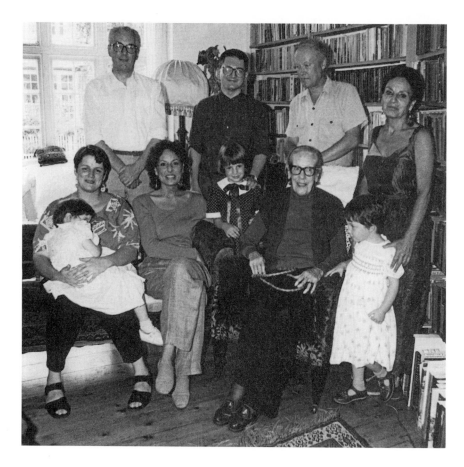

A ninetieth birthday party with four generations present – quite a common event nowadays. Each generation poses different medical problems, and in this chapter we highlight the most important of these, beginning with the deceptively simple question: why do we get old?

Age and disease

■ CONTENTS

When you look at a patient in your ward or clinic, you make a mental assessment of whether he or she is old or not. To some extent, the decision will be relative to your own age, but few will have difficulty deciding that the patient in the geriatric ward is old and the one in the neonatal ward is young! Nevertheless, to define ageing is not so easy. The reason is that, during ageing, a huge number of different variables change, ranging from purely physical characteristics to cellular and molecular changes within the cells. In general, there is a progressive deterioration in the structure and function of the body. Assuming that ageing is to do with this relentless decline, the question is: *why* do these changes occur?

THEORIES OF AGEING

A number of theories have been put forward to explain ageing. What is clear is that ageing is a multifactorial process and almost certainly involves an interaction of an internal genetic programme with external influences which damage the vital DNA machinery in the cells.

The Hayflick phenomenon

In 1961, Hayflick and his colleague Moorhead reported that normal human fibroblasts have a built-in limit to how many times they will proliferate. They suggested that these cells will multiply approximately 50 times and then stop dividing. This is known as the Hayflick limit. This observation has been extended to the whole body, and the suggestion is that all cells in the body have a limited and fixed proliferative capacity which is controlled by the cell's DNA. Exactly which bit of the DNA is involved in keeping count is unclear. Once the cell's capacity for division is lost, the cells in that particular organ cannot be replaced, which contributes to the decline of the organ's function.

The telomere hypothesis

The telomeres are bits of DNA that cap the ends of the chromosomes – rather like the metal tips on shoelaces. It has been recognized that with each cell division, part of the telomere is lost. Embryonic cells and tumour cells, however, are able to maintain their telomere length, and these cells also have the capacity to divide indefinitely. It has therefore been proposed that the telomeres act as the 'clock'. When the telomeres have been lost completely, the cells stop dividing. This idea is very plausible and may well explain some of the features of ageing. However, there are cells within our body that do not divide. These include the brain and heart muscle, but we do not die in youth because of their lack of cell division. So the telomere hypothesis cannot be the whole answer.

The free radical hypothesis

Above we have considered the theories dealing with internal genetic problems. The free radical theory relates to damage occurring from outside sources. It postulates that damage to DNA occurs as a result of free oxygen radicals being produced in the cell by environmental agents such as ionizing radiation or carcinogens. These free radicals are constantly bombarding our DNA. Although cells are initially capable of repairing the damage, with time the damage overwhelms the repair mechanisms and leads to a deterioration in the cellular DNA and hence in its function.

This free radical hypothesis has gained further favour because it has been shown that, with age, mitochondrial DNA accumulates mutations. The mitochondria are the power source for the cell, and damage to DNA here will ultimately destroy the vital energy store. This will have profound effects on the cell's ability to maintain its genome.

The glycosylation theory

Yet another hypothesis suggests that glycosylation of protein occurs progessively with ageing. This refers to the addition of sugar molecules to the proteins which allows them to crosslink, thus altering their function. This type of event is believed to underlie the microvascular disease and the cataract formation seen in diabetes (where there is excessive blood sugar). Cataracts and vascular disease are of course also a feature of old age in non-diabetics too.

You can see from this brief review that although we all understand instinctively what is meant by ageing, at the biological level it is a complex and ill-understood process. There is considerable research under way, promising new insights into the process by which we inevitably move toward deterioration and death. The understanding of ageing is tied in with our desire for longevity. At present the limit appears to be about 120 years. In another 20 years, it may be higher still. Is this what we want? An ageing population is already a major problem in developed countries. The quest for further longevity will bring with it serious ethical, social, and medical problems.

A review of the health problems/diseases commonly encountered in different age groups is shown in Boxes 13.1 to 13.4. These are not intended to be comprehensive.

■ **BOX 13.1 Neonates/children**

The main body systems of babies are evaluated at birth (1–5 minutes of age) using an APGAR score which is based on heart rate, respiration, muscle tone, response to catheter in nostril, and colour. This has been shown to be an excellent predictor of perinatal morbidity.

Accidents: Babies can be dropped or fall over; being inquisitive and fearless, they put objects into their mouths, fingers into bottles, etc; main result is cuts and bruises.

Cardiac: 'Hole in the heart': hole in septum between the two ventricles (ventricular septal defect) or auricles (atrial septal defect); patent ductus arteriosus.

Other congenital malformations: Turner's syndrome – lack of all or part of an X chromosome, leading to hypogonadism, infertility, and often heart disease; Down's syndrome – commonest of the chromosome abnormalities: trisomy of chromosome 21, mental retardation (Chapter 1); lip (hare lip) and/or palate abnormalities (cleft palate), frequently associated with chr. 13 and 18 abnormalities; congenital deficiencies of the immune system, e.g. absent thymus (DiGeorge syndrome), no B cells (Bruton's agammaglobulinaemia), complement defects, and phagocytic defects (Chapter 7). In some cases, the individual gene defects responsible for these primary immunodeficiencies have been identified.

Dermatological: Eczema – irritant dermatitis (nappy rash); asthma – mainly allergic (type I hypersensitivity, Chapter 7).

Gastrointestinal tract: Atresia – incomplete formation of oesophagus; pyloric stenosis – partial blocking of oesophagus resulting in regurgitation and persistent projectile vomiting; cow's milk intolerance.

Inborn errors of metabolism: Enzyme deficiencies: Gaucher's disease – glycocerebrosides accumulate in phagocytes; Hurler syndrome – accumulation of mucopolysaccharides, especially in phagocytes; child may develop hepatosplenomegaly; phenylketonuria – phenylalanine not converted to tyrosine; commonly tested for in urine at birth; build-up leads to brain damage.

Infections: In utero: HIV, CMV, hepatitis B; ex utero: Strep B, acquired while passing through birth canal; early childhood: measles, chickenpox, mumps, etc.

Intrauterine growth retardation: About a third of babies born are underweight owing to genetic and/or maternal factors (e.g. fetal blood supply).

Malignancy: Rare, e.g. leukaemias, Wilms' tumour of kidney.

Nutritional: Kwashiorkor – protein undernourishment; marasmus – lack of protein and carbohydrate, starvation; rickets – vitamin D deficiency – can result in leg bowing, pigeon chest, and other skeletal defects.

Respiratory: Respiratory distress syndrome – one of the most common and life-threatening conditions, also called hyaline membrane disease, due to a deficiency in a surfactant which can result in lung collapse; sudden infant death syndrome ('cot death'), associated with respiratory diseases but cause unknown.

■ BOX 13.2 Adolescents/young adults

Accidents: Bicycle, motorbike and car accidents commonest at this age.

Cardiac: Cardiomyopathies (heart muscle disease) become apparent at this age (Chapter 11).

Developmental: Growth – excessive or defective growth spurts recognized (hormonal problems associated with puberty, growth factor deficiencies).

Gastrointestinal tract: Inflammatory bowel disease (Crohn's disease and ulcerative colitis may have an immune basis).

Dermatological: Acne – males more affected than females, probably related to androgens, infections, and unknown factors; urticaria (hives) – weals produced by localized mast cell degranulation mediated by immune and non-immune mechanisms; verrucas (warts) – caused by papillomaviruses.

Malignancy: Acute leukaemias, lymphomas, and sarcomas (Chapter 12).

Metabolic: Insulin-dependent diabetes mellitus of autoimmune origin (type 1 diabetes; see Chapter 7).

Nutritional: Eating disorders: anorexia nervosa and bulimia.

Osteoarticular: Juvenile rheumatoid arthritis (juvenile chronic arthritis); juvenile ankylosing spondylitis (see Chapter 7).

Respiratory: Asthma (hyperreactive airways), caused by either allergic (hypersensitivity type I) or non-allergic mechanisms.

■ **BOX 13.3 Middle age (35–65)**

Accidents: Automobile, but less than young or old adult.

Autoimmune diseases: Generally more than earlier in life, e.g. systemic lupus erythematosus (especially in women), rheumatoid arthritis, myasthenia gravis, Sjögren's syndrome, diabetes, etc. (Chapter 7).

Cardiac: Myocardial infarcts are more common than cardiomyopathies.

Gastrointestinal tract: Chronic and acute peptic ulcers in stomach and duodenum; cause unknown, but *Helicobacter pylori* involved and can be treated with antibiotics. Inflammatory bowel disease also common in this age group.

Malignancy: Solid tumours – colon cancer, breast cancer; rare leukaemias.

Metabolic: Diabetes and its complications, including kidney, eye, and vascular; complications usually due to small vessel aneurysms.

Osteoarticular: Osteoarthritis, rheumatoid arthritis, and ankylosing spondylitis; bone resorption as the result of Paget's disease.

Respiratory: Infections, may be associated with smoking.

■ **BOX 13.4 Old age (65+)**

Accidents: Falls resulting in fractures which are slower to heal at this age, as are wounds in general.

Cardiac: Myocardial infarcts, aneurysms (atheromatous – Chapter 11)

Central nervous system: Dementias, strokes (Chapter 11).

Infection: Commoner as the function of the immune system decreases.

Degenerative: Osteoarthritis, general immobility as a result of muscle/tendon degeneration.

Malignancy: Solid tumours, breast, prostate, and lung carcinomas; chronic leukaemias, e.g. CLL (Chapter 12).

Nutritional: Malnutrion due to social deprivation, absorption problems.

Osteoarticular: Osteoarthritis; osteoporosis – can be exacerbated in menopausal women; osteomalacia–undermineralization of bone, some due to lack of dietary vitamin D but most due to secondary causes, e.g. chronic renal disease.

Respiratory: Chronic obstructive airways disease (COAD), general term for chronic bronchitis, emphysema, asthma, and bronchiectasis – increased incidence with heavy smoking.

Social: Hypothermia; psychiatric (especially depression).

Tutorial 13

Here is a short test of your 'feel' for what conditions are common at different ages.

QUESTIONS

Name five pathological problems that are likely to occur in:

1. A newborn baby.

2. A 10-year-old boy.

3. A 25-year-old woman.

4. A 50-year-old man.

5. An 85-year-old.

ANSWERS

1. Congenital abnormalities: Down's, respiratory distress syndrome, congenital heart disease; Rhesus disease; low birth weight (intrauterine growth retardation); cerebral palsy; birth marks (haemangiomas).

2. Malignancies, e.g. leukaemias, soft tissue, germ cells; endocrine – growth increase or retardation; psychological e.g. autism (school bullying, truancy); recurrent ear infections ('glue' ear); accidents, fractures, e.g. bicycle; malabsorption – coeliac disease; asthma; diabetes (type 1).

3. Endocrine, e.g. abnormal menstrual cycles with heavy bleeding, thyrotoxicosis; cervical dysplasia (wart virus, promiscuity); rheumatoid arthritis; accidents – car; ectopic pregnancy; malignancy – leukaemia, rarely breast, ovary (familial); psychiatric – anorexia, bulimia.

4. Myocardial infarction; peptic and duodenal ulcer; tumours, e.g. lymphoma, GI tract; respiratory – chronic obstructive airways diseases; diabetes – adult onset non-insulin-dependent diabetes; renal – related to increased blood pressure; pancreas/liver – alcohol.

5. Cerebrovascular accidents, e.g. strokes; myocardial infarction; falls leading to fracture; osteoporosis; osteoarthritis; hypothermia; malnutrition; accidents – burns.

FURTHER READING

Cotton D 1996. Ageing and death. In: Underwood J C E (ed), General and systemic pathology, 2nd edn. Churchill Livingstone, Edinburgh, 941 pp

Hayflick L 1996 How and why we age. Ballantine Books, New York, 377 pp

Selkoe D 1992. Aging brain, aging mind. Scientific American (special issue), September, pp 96–103

Shatz C 1992. The developing brain. Scientific American (special issue), September, pp 34–41

Terminology of inflammatory disease

The terminology of inflammatory disease is usually self-explanatory, but there are exceptions. The most commonly met terms are shown below, with some examples of their use.

Term	Meaning		Comments
Adenitis	Inflammation of a gland		e.g. lymphadenitis (q.v.)
Alveolitis	"	lung alveoli	e.g. extrinsic allergic
Aortitis	"	aorta	
Appendicitis	"	appendix	
Arteritis	"	arteries	e.g. peri-, poly-
Arthritis	"	joints	e.g. osteo-, rheumatoid
Bronchitis	"	bronchi	
Bursitis	"	bursa(e)	e.g. tennis elbow
Cellulitis	Spreading inflammation in deep tissues		
Cholangitis	Inflammation of bile duct		
Cholecystitis	"	gallbladder	
Colitis	"	colon	e.g. ulcerative
Cystitis	"	bladder	
Dermatitis	"	skin	e.g. contact, atopic
Dermatomyositis	"	skin and muscle	
Diverticulitis	"	diverticula	Usually in colon
Encephalitis	"	brain and/or spinal cord	
Endocarditis	"	inner lining of heart	
Enteritis	"	intestine	Often with stomach (gastro-)
Epiglottitis	"	epiglottis	
Fibrositis	Unexplained localized muscular pain and tenderness		
Folliculitis	Inflammation of hair follicles		
Gastritis	"	stomach	See also enteritis
Glomerulonephritis	"	kidney	Often called 'nephritis'
Hepatitis	"	liver	
Ileitis	"	ileum	Often with colitis
Iridocyclitis	"	iris and ciliary body of eye	
Keratitis	"	cornea	
Laryngitis	"	larynx	*(cont'd)*

Term	Meaning		Comments
Lymphadenitis	Inflammation of lymph glands		
Lymphangitis	"	lymphatics	
Mastitis	"	breast	
Meningitis	"	meninges (of brain)	
Myocarditis	"	heart muscle	
Myositis	"	skeletal muscle	
Nephritis	"	kidney	See also glomerulonephritis
Neuritis	"	nerves	e.g. poly-, peripheral
Oesophagitis	"	oesophagus	
Oophoritis	"	ovary	
Ophthalmitis	"	eye	e.g. sympathetic
Orchitis	"	testis	
Osteomyelitis	"	bone (strictly, bone marrow)	
Otitis	"	ear	e.g. -media (middle ear)
Pancreatitis	"	pancreas	
Parotitis	"	parotid gland	e.g. mumps
Pericarditis	"	pericardium	
Peritonitis	"	peritoneum	
Pharyngitis	"	pharynx	
Phlebitis	"	veins	Also thrombo-
Pneumonia	"	lung	Including air spaces
Pneumonitis	"	lung	Excluding pneumonia
Poliomyelitis	"	brain and spinal cord, caused by poliovirus	
Poly-	"	multiple sites (e.g. polyarthritis)	
Proctitis	"	rectum	
Prostatitis	"	prostate	
Pyelonephritis	"	renal pelvis	Bacterial only
Retinitis	"	retina (of eye)	
Rhinitis	"	nose	e.g. allergic
Salpingitis	"	fallopian tubes	
Sinusitis	"	nasal sinuses	
Spondylitis	"	spinal joints	e.g. ankylosing
Stomatitis	"	mouth	
Tenosynovitis	"	tendon sheaths	
Thyroiditis	"	thyroid	
Tonsillitis	"	tonsils	
Tracheitis	"	trachea	Also tracheobronchitis
Urethritis	"	urethra	
Uveitis	"	uveal tract of eye	
Vasculitis	"	blood vessels	

Categorization of biological agents according to hazard and categories of containment

Type of agent	Category 4 (P 4): severe disease; no treatment; maximum isolation and security	Category 3 (P 3): serious disease; vaccine or treatment available; separate restricted facility	Category 2 (P 2): vaccine or treatment available; unlikely to spread; safety cabinet
Virus	Lassa Ebola Marburg Smallpox	Dengue Hepatitis B, C, D, E HIV Rabies Yellow fever (Prions)	Hepatitis A Herpes 1–7 Influenza Measles Mumps Polio Rubella
Bacterium		Anthrax Brucella Mycobacterium Rickettsia Salmonella[1] Shigella[1] Plague	Bordetella pertussis Campylobacter Tetanus Diphtheria E. coli Haemophilus Legionella Listeria Gonococcus Meningococcus Pseudomonas Staphylococcus Streptococcus Vibrio (cholera)
Fungus		Blastomyces Histoplasma	Aspergillus Candida
Protozoon		Leishmania[1] Plasmodium Trypanosoma	Amoeba Giardia Toxoplasma
Worm		Echinococcus	Hookworm Schistosoma

[1]Only the most virulent species; the remainder are Category 2.

Autopsy

The number of autopsies (postmortem examinations, PMs) has been declining in this country for the last 30 years, and many teaching hospitals perform less than 100 autopsies each year, an average of less than 2 per week. Autopsy was one of the principal sources of material for medical education in the past. It also has a role in clinical audit, since, despite the advances in technology, autopsies regularly turn up pathological conditions unsuspected during life.

Paramedical staff, particularly nurses who have direct contact with patients and their relatives, are often in a position to influence their decision regarding consent for the examination. However, not everyone understands the legal background to the process of consent. Further, the value of autopsy in teaching, audit, and research is often unclear.

THE CORONER'S AUTOPSY

A coroner is appointed by local or central government and is usually a doctor or a lawyer or both. The coroner's job is to enquire into deaths which have unnatural, suspicious, or criminal aspects. The coroner's autopsy is therefore a legal requirement. In this situation, a death certificate cannot be issued until the autopsy has been performed.

Some of the reasons for reporting a death to the coroner are listed below:

- The body is unidentified.
- No doctor has attended the person during the last illness.
- It is not possible to certify the death as due to natural causes.
- Death occurred during an operation or before the patient recovered from an anaesthetic.
- Sudden death under suspicious circumstances.
- Death related to violence or accident.
- Death linked with an abortion.
- Death due to an industrial disease.
- Death possibly due to lack of medical care.

There are a number of other reasons, and full details can be obtained from autopsy handbooks or legal textbooks. When in doubt, the doctor should always discuss the case with the coroner before issuing a death certificate.

THE HOSPITAL AUTOPSY

In contrast, the hospital autopsy is requested *after* the death certificate has been issued. The doctor can only issue the death certificate without referring to the coroner if:

- He has attended the patient during the last illness.
- He has seen the patient in the last 14 days prior to death.
- He knows the cause of death (or, more realistically, thinks that he knows the cause of death).
- He is satisfied that the death is wholly due to natural causes.

Having issued the death certificate stating the cause of death, the doctor may then request a postmortem by obtaining consent from the relatives. The relatives may consent to the whole autopsy, a limited autopsy looking at a particular site or organ, or an autopsy in which consent is *not* given for tissue to be saved for research or to teach students. The relatives often find it difficult to comprehend why an autopsy is necessary when the cause of death is already known. In fact there are a number of reasons why this may be important:

- To confirm the clinical evidence for audit (i.e. the evaluation of the accuracy and efficiency of the medical service).
- To assess other pathological conditions which may be important for future reference but which did not directly contribute to the patient's death.
- To correlate the data derived from new technologies (e.g. MRI imaging) with histological diagnosis.
- To assess the toxic effects of new or experimental drugs.

PRINCIPAL BENEFITS

The principal benefits are:

- For the patient's relatives: obtaining details of the disease process and confirmation of the cause of death.
- For the doctor looking after the patient: confirmation of the cause of death, an understanding of the clinical problem at the tissue level, identification of pathology not apparent clinically.
- For the students: a chance to learn pathology, which forms the core science of medical education, directly from real human beings rather than from fixed and preserved specimens.
- For the hospital: ability to carry out audit on the quality of care of patients within the institution.

FURTHER READING

Cotton D N K, Cross 1993 The hospital autopsy. Butterworth-Heinemann, Oxford

Knight B 1983 The coroner's autopsy. Churchill Livingstone, Edinburgh

Commonly requested tests

Here are some blood and urine tests you will often hear being requested from the pathology departments, together with a guide to the normal range of values. Note that these may vary slightly from hospital to hospital, depending on the exact technique in use.

Sample	Normal range
Blood	
Haemoglobin	13–17 g/DL (male); 11.5–15.5 g/DL (female)
Red cells	4.4–5.8 × 10^{12}/L (male); 3.95–5.15 (female)
White cells (total)	4–11 × 10^9/L
Neutrophils (PMN)	2–7.5 × 10^9/L (40–75%)
Lymphocytes (total)	1.5–4 × 10^9 (20–45%)
B cells	0.05–0.6 × 10^9/L
T cells, CD4	0.35–2.2 × 10^9/L
CD8	0.2–1.5 × 10^9/L
Platelets	150–400 × 10^9/L
Sedimentation rate (ESR)	1–20 mm/h
Plasma	
Glucose	3.3–5.6 mmol/L (fasting)
Sodium	137–145 mmol/L
Potassium	3.3–4.8 mmol/L
Calcium	2.2–2.6 mmol/L
Bicarbonate	20–30 mmol/L
Albumin	35–53 g/L
Cholesterol	2.3–6.9 mmol/L
Urea	3–8 mmol/L
Complement; C3	0.75–1.75 g/L
Immunoglobulins; IgG	8–18 g/L
IgA	0.9–4.5 g/L
IgM	0.6–2.8 g/L
IgE	0.3 mg/L
Urine	
Glucose	0–0.3 mmol/L (fasting)
Protein	0–0.1 g/24 h

Glossary

Abscess	Localized collection of pus
Adenocarcinoma	Malignant tumour of glandular epithelium
Adenoma	Benign tumour of glandular epithelium
Adjuvant	A substance which non-specifically enhances the immune response to an antigen (e.g. alum given with vaccines)
Aetiology	The cause of the disease
Agenesis	Failure of tissue to form during embryogensis
Allele	One of the two copies of a particular gene. Each copy (allele) is derived from one of the parents
Allergy	Type I (IgE-mediated) hypersensitivity
Allograft	Graft between non-identical animals of same species
Anaemia	Low haemoglobin concentration in the blood
Anaplastic	Complete lack of differentiation in a tumour
Aneurysm	Dilatation of a vessel or of the heart leading to outpouching
Anoxia	Lack of oxygen
Antibiotic	A drug used to treat microbial infection, e.g. penicillin
Antibody	A protein produced by B lymphocytes, able to bind to antigen; also known as immunoglobulin
Antigen	A molecule that induces the formation of antibody; usually a protein or carbohydrate
Apoptosis	Special type of cell death which results from cell suicide
Atheroma	Accumulation of lipids in vessels leading to damage of the wall and narrowing of lumen
Atherosclerosis	Hardening of the arteries due to atheroma
Atopy, atopic	Allergy, or the tendency to develop this

Atrophy	Decrease in cell number or size
Autograft	Graft from one site to another in same individual
Autopsy	Another name for 'postmortem'
Bacillus	A rod-shaped bacterium
Bronchiectasis	Abnormal and permanent dilatation of the bronchi
Calculus	Calcified stone formation, e.g. kidney stone, gallstone
Cancer	A malignant tumour – unspecified
Carcinogenesis	The process by which malignant tumours arise
Carcinoma	Malignant tumour of epithelial tissue
Carcinoma in situ	Malignant tumour of epithelial tissue but confined within the basement membrane
CVA	Cerebrovascular accident ('stroke')
Chemotaxis	Movement of cells along a chemical gradient
Clone	Population of cells derived from single precursor; *used of both* bacteria and lymphocytes
Coccus	A roughly spherical bacterium
Complement	A system of serum proteins involved in immunity and inflammation
Consolidation	Tissue becoming solid owing to infection, e.g. pneumonia
Cyst	Cavity containing fluid and lined by epithelium
Differentiation	Process of acquiring specialized function in cells or tissues. In tumour pathology, it refers to how closely the tumour resembles the normal tissue
Dysplasia	Morphological and cytological abnormality seen in tissue and believed to have premalignant connotations
Ectopic	Tissue in a site away from its normal position, e.g. ectopic pregnancy occurring in the fallopian tube
Effusion	Collection of fluid in a body cavity, e.g. pleural effusion
Embolus	A mass of tissue or gas that moves from one place to another in the circulation
Fibrosis	Deposition of collagen in tissues

Fistula	An abnormal connection between two hollow structures (e.g. bowel to bowel) or between hollow structure and skin
Gangrene	Dead necrotic tissue with black appearance; may be sterile ('dry') or infected ('wet')
Grade	An assessment of how closely or little the tumour resembles the parent tissue
Granulation tissue	New connective tissue, new blood vessels and inflammatory cells, formed at edge of healing wounds and ulcers
Granuloma	A collection of macrophages sometimes surrounded by lymphocytes
Histogenesis	Cellular origin of a particular cell or tissue
Humoral	In blood or tissue fluid, e.g. antibody ('humoral') response
Hyperplasia	Increase in cell number
Hypersensitivity	Tissue-damaging immune response, e.g. type I, II, etc.
Hypertrophy	Increase in cell size
Hypoxia	Decreased oxygen tension in tissues
Immune complex	Antibody combined with antigen; may cause tissue damage ('immune complex disease')
Infarction	Death of tissue due to lack of adequate blood supply
Involution	Decrease in size of an organ
Ischaemia	Decrease in blood supply to an organ or tissue
Leukaemia	Malignant tumour of white blood cells
Lymphoma	Malignant tumour of lymphoid tissue
Metaplasia	Reversible change of one type of normal epithelium to another
Metastasis	Tumour spread to sites away from the site of origin
Mitosis	Cell division
Monoclonal antibody	Antibody produced by single clone of B cells and therefore of a single specificity
Mutation	Alteration in the DNA sequence which may lead to abnormal protein production
Necrosis	Cell or tissue death

Neoplasm	Literally 'new growth'. In tumours it implies an autonomous growth which has escaped regulatory mechanisms
Oncogene	Any mutated gene which leads to neoplastic transformation
Opportunist	A microbe that only causes disease in immunodeficient patients
Opsonin	A molecule that enhances the phagoctosis of ('opsonizes') a microbe, e.g. antibody, complement
Organization	Process of tissue repair with some residual fibrosis or scar formation
Passive immunity	Immunity conferred by injecting preformed antibody
Pathogenesis	The pathological process from cause (aetiology) to clinical manifestation
Phagocytosis	Ingestion of material (debris, microbes) by cells
Pleomorphism	Variation in size and shape – usually refers to nuclei
Polyp	Pedunculated growth, e.g. in colon
Polyposis	Multiple polyps
Pus	Composed of dead and dying bacteria, white blood cells (polymorphs), and cells from the tissue
Regeneration	Replacement of dead tissue by replicating new cells
Repair	Replacement of dead tissue either by scar tissue or by local replication of cells
Sarcoma	Malignant tumour of connective tissue
Septic	Infected
Septicaemia	Infection in the bloodstream, usually bacterial
Shock	Cardiovascular collapse, e.g. due to blood loss or septicaemia
Teratoma	Germ cell tumour containing mixture of tissues (epithelial, connective tissue, neural etc.) Found in testis and ovary
Thrombus	Mass of coagulated blood within the circulation
Toxoid	Inactivated toxin used as vaccine
Vaccine	Microbial preparation used to induce immunity
Xenograft	Graft between animals of different species

Index

D